The Complete Guide to Modern Massage

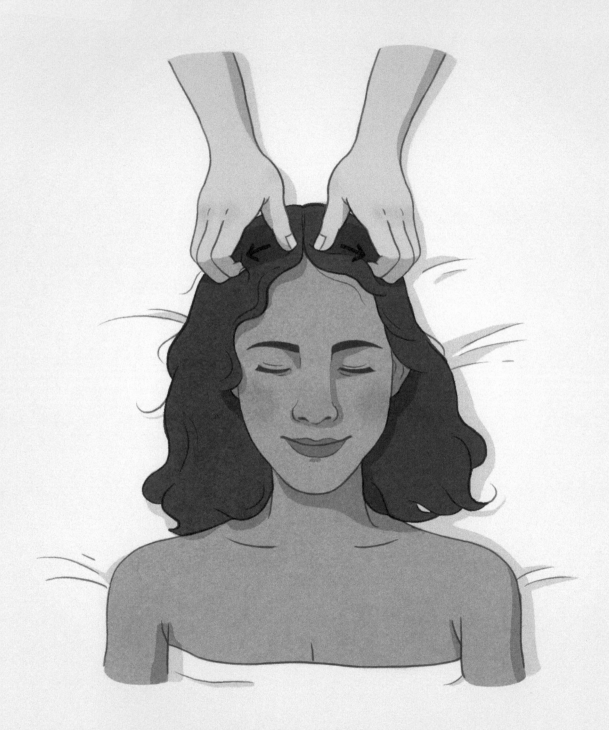

The Complete Guide to

Modern Massage

Step-by-Step Massage Basics and Techniques from Around the World

RYAN JAY HOYME, LMT, BCTMB

ALTHEA PRESS

Interior Designer: Liz Cosgrove
Cover Designer: Amy King
Editor: Melissa Valentine
Production Editor: Andrew Yackira
Illustrations © Christy Ni, 2018;
page 110: Peter Hermes Furian/Shutterstock.com
Cover photography © Trinette Reed/Blend Images
Author photo © Alexa Hoyme, 2018.

ISBN: Print 978-1-64152-206-9
eBook 978-1-64152-207-6

In memory of my beloved little sister,
Beth Ann

Contents

3: Techniques for the Whole Body   33

4: Techniques from Around the World   65

Introduction

Massage has many widely known benefits including relaxation, pain relief, and stress reduction. But I admit that my first experience with massage was . . . less than pleasant. I never would have guessed that I would go on to become a licensed massage therapist and teacher known as the Massage Nerd.

For that first massage, when I was 21, I went to a Chinese Medicine practitioner for a back injury. He performed fire cupping (using glass cups that are heated inside and then quickly placed on the body) and barefoot massage (where the practitioner holds onto a beam to support his weight while using his feet to massage the client). I'd never even heard of those techniques and at no point did he explain to me what he was doing! I did start to feel a little better after the treatment, but the sense of surprise and lack of communication didn't make me eager to go back. Even still, the relief I felt was undeniable and soon, another injury would lead me back to the massage table.

I was reintroduced to massage after I injured myself while helping lift patients in the nursing home where I was working. I made some appointments to see a physical therapist, but after months of doing stretches and exercises, nothing seemed to help. Then the physical therapist started to incorporate massage therapy into our sessions and I only then started to feel better. I've been hooked ever since. In fact, the healing benefits were so profound, I decided to pivot my career and study massage. I enrolled in a massage program the following month. After I completed my schooling, I worked as a massage therapist in a health club, and eventually in private practice. I was working toward running my own massage business full-time when I got a call from somebody asking if I'd be interested in teaching massage therapy. I was shocked because I'd never spoken in front of people before, let alone taught—just the thought of it made me break out in a sweat. But I decided to give it a go and I'm so glad I did. I've taught thousands of students over the years, and while they learned a lot from me, I believe I learned so much more from them. I learned about passion, perseverance, and resolve. I came to understand that people learn at different paces and in different ways. And, perhaps most importantly, I learned about the power of visual teaching.

During my 12-year teaching career I noticed that most massage books didn't show a wide enough range of techniques. After the first class I taught, I decided to draw my methods and give them to my students. I can't draw to save my life, and the students laughed at the illustrations, but they were still always using my manual. I noticed that some students needed a little more help, so I started creating videos of my techniques. Back then in 2006, most massage therapists were not recording their massage techniques. Videos were one of the main things that helped me get known in the massage profession, and I owe this to my students.

Around that time, a student called me a "massage nerd," and something clicked. I immediately bought the domain MassageNerd.com. Over the years I've shot over 5,000 videos and grown a dedicated following on my YouTube channel. I've been a massage therapist for 21 years and while I'm no longer actively teaching, I continue to educate people through my website and social media. Teaching massage is my passion, and it's an honor to share this knowledge with you.

There are over 200 different styles of massage, and it can get a little confusing to decipher how the methods differ and which is best for you. Most of the techniques in this book are Western-based (Swedish massage), but many are influenced by other methods from around the world, including Thai massage, Tui na massage (Chinese), Shiatsu (Japanese), and more.

In the first part of this book, I walk you through the history of massage, the mind-body connection, and basic anatomy, providing you with the foundation you need for giving and receiving massage. From there, I offer massage techniques for the whole body complete with step-by-step instructions and helpful illustrations. I also share instructions for my favorite styles from around the world; positions and techniques for special life circumstances, such as prenatal, baby, couples, and senior massage; and special healing techniques for pain. When starting any new program, such as the massage techniques presented in this book, always consult your physician or other healthcare professional. The information in this book is not intended to diagnose or cure any medical condition or to replace your healthcare professional. Consult with your healthcare professional if you have any concerns about any of the techniques in this book. If you experience any pain or difficulty with any technique, stop and consult your healthcare provider immediately.

The main thing I'd like you to get from reading this is that that you need a strong foundation before you go to the next level with your practice. For that reason, I suggest reading the book from beginning to end, trying the different massage techniques and finding out what works for you. Once you're more confident, you can combine the different methods to establish your own unique style. I'm a firm believer that *anyone* can perform massage so I've intentionally written this book for all levels. It's for the beginner home practitioner who wants to give massages to friends, relatives, and partners, as well as for the aspiring or practicing massage therapist looking to learn new techniques and brush up their knowledge; it also is a great gift—just be sure you get a massage in return!

CHAPTER 1

Massage

The body is an incredibly complex system. Massage meets this system at the skin somewhere between anatomy, kinesiology, and medicine. The skin is the first access point to the body and all its complex parts—the vital organs, bones, muscles, and fascia—where we have the unique human ability to literally heal with our hands. You don't have to be a professional to be able to give a great massage, but it's useful to know as much as you can about the human body in order to help people reap the most benefits.

The Importance of Touch

Touch is one of the most basic human needs, yet it's often neglected. Your skin receives the sense of touch through nerve endings all over your body, and this sensation has been shown to aid in physical and emotional health. An infant craves touch when they're born—it's an instinctive desire and way of communicating love, nurturance, trust, caring, comfort, safety, and more. When we're adults, that desire and ability to communicate through touch doesn't go away. It's still very much a necessary part of relating to and healing one another. It's no surprise, then, that massage can invoke emotional responses like tears of joy and a feeling of relief. Touch has the power to awaken and release emotions stored in the body.

THE SCIENCE OF TOUCH

Massage takes the benefits of physical connection to the next level. In fact, massage has been shown to increase oxytocin, the hormone that regulates positive emotions and social interactions, and to reduce the adrenocorticotropic hormone, which stimulates the release of cortisol (the "stress hormone"). The takeaway? Touch in the form of massage has many benefits, and it can help you physically *and* emotionally.

The History of Massage

The history of massage goes back as long as humans have been on this planet. Just think about it: If you're in pain, you'll touch that area and instinctively start massaging it. The earliest written records of massage were found in China, Egypt, and India dating back thousands of years. Unfortunately there hasn't been a lot of history recorded about massage, and the dates can be conflicting, but here's an abbreviated timeline of what we do know:

BCE 2330: The Egyptian Tomb of Akmanthor, also known as "The Tomb of the Physician," shows two men touching each other's feet and hands.

BCE 1800: The oldest written record of massage is around 4,000 years old and was found in an ancient Chinese medical text, *Con-Fu of the Toa-Tse.* The text mentioned application of massage techniques.

BCE 460: Hippocrates wrote: "The physician must be experienced in many things, but assuredly in rubbing." This shows how thousands of years ago, touch was a method that physicians used regularly because they didn't have the technology we have today to diagnose and treat pain. The more the medical system advances, the less it relies on touch.

1700–1800s: Pehr Henrik Ling (1776–1839), a Swedish physical therapist and teacher of medical gymnastics, is credited for having invented "Classic massage" (also known as Swedish Massage). He's often called the "Father of Massage."

1800s: Johann Georg Mezger (1838–1909) is credited with developing the terms effleurage (gliding), petrissage (squeezing or kneading), friction (pressing), tapotement (percussion), and vibration (shaking).

1943: The first professional massage association, American Massage Therapy Association, was formed.

1992: The National Certification Board for Therapeutic Massage & Bodywork was founded. This was a watershed moment for massage because it was the first national certification for massage therapists. Now massage therapists can become board certified, which is the highest credential in the massage profession.

Early 2010s: This era saw a huge surge in massage schools popping up, even in some colleges. This made training a lot more accessible.

Modern Massage

Massage as a field and healing practice has come a long way since I began my studies. There were many things we were told we had to be cautious of when giving massages. For example, we were told we could not massage people with cancer because it would increase the cancer cells in the body. This is one misconception about massage that has been debunked. I routinely massage people with cancer in the hospital where I work; however, there are still precautions, so you must be trained in oncology massage. We were also warned against massaging pregnant women in their first trimester. Most experts in the prenatal massage field now say this is okay, as long as it is not a high-risk pregnancy. (And once again, you need proper training in prenatal massage.)

There has been an even bigger shift in perception recently. Massage was once widely considered a luxury, meant only for those who could afford fancy spa days. Now it's accepted as part of a healthy lifestyle, and an important healing and self-care practice. You can now find massage therapists in most health clubs, chiropractic offices, wellness centers, spas, hotels and cruise ships, and at private practices. Most hospitals, such as the one I work at, now offer massage therapy to patients. The areas I work in include the birthing center, mental health, medical surgical, ambulatory surgery, and outpatient.

Today, more and more people want to learn massage—either to help friends and family, learn how to work on themselves, or to start their own career in massage. Now that its healing benefits are widely known, more people want to learn how to give a massage at home.

Massage has become so much more accessible over the years. For example, massage products have gotten a lot cheaper. Back in 1997, I paid over $500 for a basic massage table—now you can buy one for around $100. Massage supplies are generally more widely available (see chapter two, beginning on page 19, for suggestions on tools and materials).

When it comes to massage techniques, there is so much variety. And as you will find out in the upcoming chapters, many massage techniques overlap. In modern massage, it's rare to stick to just one style. It's much more common for practitioners to blend different techniques from other styles and make it their own. This book provides the foundation to help you eventually build your own unique style as well.

East & West

For many years, Eastern and Western massage—for instance, Thai massage compared with Swedish massage—were separate. But today, these styles are commonly blended. Western massage therapists are starting to take bits and pieces of Eastern massage and make it their own.

EASTERN MASSAGE

Rooted in Eastern medicine, where the body is treated as one unified system including the mind and spirit, this type of massage focuses on flow and balance of energy within the body. The techniques are meant to relax specific points in order to help the vital energy flow. Eastern-influenced massage therapists figure out where to focus on the body by determining where energy imbalances lie, and not necessarily the area of discomfort.

WESTERN MASSAGE

Western massage is rooted in Western medicine, which separates the parts of the body by their function. This massage style (commonly referred to as Swedish massage) tends to focus on the individual parts of the body where pain or discomfort lie. Massage therapists of this style will use massage techniques on or around the painful areas.

The real separation that still rings true today is that Eastern massage is more based on acupressure points, meridian lines and in Thai massage, sen lines. Western massage is more based on trigger point therapy. However, a lot of the trigger points and acupressure points do overlap.

Trigger Points

A trigger point is a sensitive knot found within bands of skeletal muscles. They can occur for a number of reasons including, injury, trauma, or basic strain. These sore spots cause pain and limit range of motion in the body. There are hundreds of trigger points on the body. Some massage therapists say that if you are treating only the painful area, you're in the wrong area 75 percent of the time. For example, most headaches start in the neck or shoulders but refer pain to the head. If you want to be good at determining the possible source of pain, it's important to know the trigger points on the body, and where the possible referrals may be.

Touching a trigger point stimulates activity in a sensory neuron, which then passes to the part of the brain that's associated with that body location. It's an instant feeling that can have huge rewards for your body, mind, and spirit.

BENEATH THE SURFACE

The more you can relax the muscles with massage, the more likely the skin, fascia, and organs can relax, too. There's also been a lot of positive research on the effectiveness of massage for lowering inflammation. Additionally, massage is now widely used to help with the following ailments:

- Symptoms of fibromyalgia
- Pain in cancer patients
- Lowering blood pressure
- Post-operative pain
- Chronic neck pain
- Knee pain
- Low back pain
- Hormone and immune function

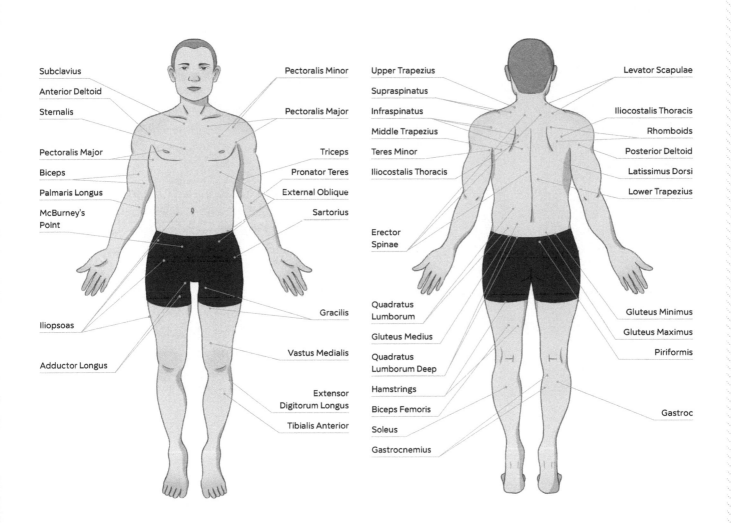

Subclavius

Anterior Deltoid

Sternalis

Pectoralis Major

Biceps

Palmaris Longus

McBurney's Point

Iliopsoas

Adductor Longus

Pectoralis Minor

Pectoralis Major

Triceps

Pronator Teres

External Oblique

Sartorius

Gracilis

Vastus Medialis

Extensor Digitorum Longus

Tibialis Anterior

Upper Trapezius

Supraspinatus

Infraspinatus

Middle Trapezius

Teres Minor

Iliocostalis Thoracis

Erector Spinae

Quadratus Lumborum

Gluteus Medius

Quadratus Lumborum Deep

Hamstrings

Biceps Femoris

Soleus

Gastrocnemius

Levator Scapulae

Iliocostalis Thoracis

Rhomboids

Posterior Deltoid

Latissimus Dorsi

Lower Trapezius

Gluteus Minimus

Gluteus Maximus

Piriformis

Gastroc

Common trigger points

Basic Anatomy for Massage

In order to begin using massage, it's important to understand anatomy basics for massage: the muscular and skeletal systems. Let's go over some basic anatomy.

> "The brain and peripheral nervous system, the endocrine and immune systems, and indeed, all the organs of our body and all the emotional responses we have, share a common chemical language and are constantly communicating with one another."
>
> ~ Dr. James Gordon
> (Center for Mind-Body Medicine)

THE SKELETAL AND MUSCULAR SYSTEMS

The muscular system is the primary body system that you'll need to know on your massage journey; however, a basic understanding of the skeletal systems will give you a more complete picture of the body and how it functions in the context of massage. It's all interconnected.

Muscular system: There are around 650 muscles in the human body. There are three types of muscles: smooth, cardiac, and skeletal muscles. They help with movement, move substances through organs, and help pump blood. During a massage, you'll be working with skeletal muscles.

Skeletal system: The adult human has 206 bones, as well as a network of tendons, ligaments, and cartilage. This skeletal system helps with movement of the body, production of blood cells, and storage of calcium.

FASCIA

As we move through the body systems, we're getting closer and closer to the body's surface, the access point of massage. When we give a massage, we're working primarily with skeletal muscles and fascia, the tissue that surrounds them. Fascia is a form of connective tissue. If you've even received a professional massage or seen a physical therapist, you may have heard this word before. It is a thin sheath of fibrous tissue enclosing muscles, bones, and organs throughout the entire body. Massage reduces tension of the fascia and the muscles it surrounds, creating greater range of motion, reducing tightness, and generating better flow and function to the fascia itself and to the surrounding body systems.

There are three layers of fascia:

1. **Superficial fascia** is the lowermost layer of the skin in nearly all of the regions of the body that blends with the reticular dermis layer, or skin. The majority of myofascial release techniques (page 123) focus on this layer of the fascia.

2. **Visceral fascia** (also called subserous fascia) supports the organs within their cavities and wraps them in layers of connective tissue membranes. Each organ is covered in a double layer of fascia, and thin serous membranes separate them. This layer is harder to access through massage.

3. **Deep fascia** is a layer of dense fibrous connective tissue, which surrounds individual muscles, and divides groups of muscles. By increasing pressure, you can access this layer through massage techniques.

When your muscles are tight, the surrounding fascia tightens along with them. Over time the fascia becomes tight, and can compress the muscles and the nerves by restricting blood flow and movement. The more relaxed fascia is, the more flexible your muscles and nerves will be.

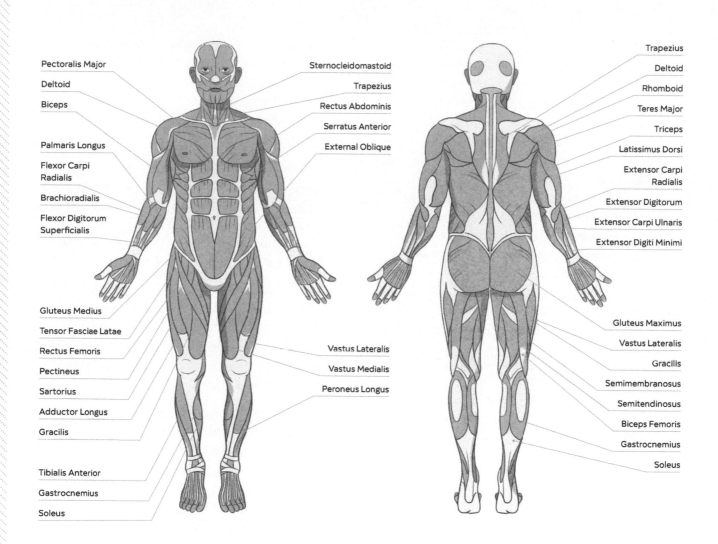

Pectoralis Major

Deltoid

Biceps

Palmaris Longus

Flexor Carpi Radialis

Brachioradialis

Flexor Digitorum Superficialis

Gluteus Medius

Tensor Fasciae Latae

Rectus Femoris

Pectineus

Sartorius

Adductor Longus

Gracilis

Tibialis Anterior

Gastrocnemius

Soleus

Sternocleidomastoid

Trapezius

Rectus Abdominis

Serratus Anterior

External Oblique

Vastus Lateralis

Vastus Medialis

Peroneus Longus

Trapezius

Deltoid

Rhomboid

Teres Major

Triceps

Latissimus Dorsi

Extensor Carpi Radialis

Extensor Digitorum

Extensor Carpi Ulnaris

Extensor Digiti Minimi

Gluteus Maximus

Vastus Lateralis

Gracilis

Semimembranosus

Semitendinosus

Biceps Femoris

Gastrocnemius

Soleus

There are over 600 muscles in the body. These are some of the main skeletal muscles that are targeted during massage.

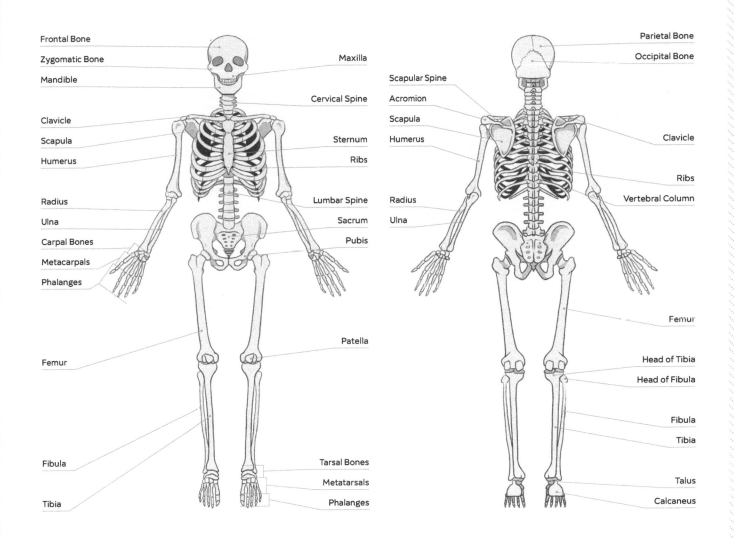

Frontal Bone
Zygomatic Bone
Mandible
Clavicle
Scapula
Humerus
Radius
Ulna
Carpal Bones
Metacarpals
Phalanges
Femur
Fibula
Tibia

Maxilla
Cervical Spine
Sternum
Ribs
Lumbar Spine
Sacrum
Pubis
Patella
Tarsal Bones
Metatarsals
Phalanges

Scapular Spine
Acromion
Scapula
Humerus
Radius
Ulna

Parietal Bone
Occipital Bone
Clavicle
Ribs
Vertebral Column
Femur
Head of Tibia
Head of Fibula
Fibula
Tibia
Talus
Calcaneus

Humans are born with nearly 300 bones, but most adults have around 206 because some bones will eventually grow together. It is important to never massage directly on a bone.

Mind-Body Connection

The mind-body connection is another system of the body so to speak, but an invisible one; it is how our thoughts, feelings, beliefs, and attitudes can affect the body and emotions. What we do with our bodies—how we eat, how we move, how much sleep we get—can change our mental state. This results in a complex interrelationship between our minds and bodies. In my own experience, I've witnessed that when the mind starts to relax, the body responds in order to absorb the full benefits of the massage. When I coach people through taking a few deep breaths and calming their mind, it usually helps induce a relaxation response in the body and makes my work easier.

Energy healing takes this concept even further. It is an aspect of many massage modalities that use energetic and emotional systems to aid in healing. Meridians, chakras, and other energy systems have been around a lot longer than modern medicine. Chakras and meridians are based on energy, and altering them through energy healing can affect someone spiritually, physically and emotionally. To work with chakras, the giver generally hovers over or places their hands on a specific chakra. With meridians, the giver presses or massages on the meridian lines and acupressure points. Just as touch and release of tension through muscle and fascia, with energetic methods, it's possible to release and move energy in a similar manner.

WHAT IS A KNOT?

Specific areas of tightness in the body are commonly called "knots." Knots are trigger points that cause pain or are tender to the touch. These spots are hyperirritable points in muscle tissue caused by a small fiber or group of fibers cramping or going into a spasm. These spots can cause you pain in the area, limit your range of motion, and cause the tissue to feel different—like a tight little ball.

These trigger points can be released by pressing on the tender area and bringing the pressure to about a 6 on a 1–10 scale, with 10 being the most discomfort. Press and wait for the muscle to relax around your thumbs, fingers, or palms. Once the discomfort has lessened, then you can slowly increase the pressure to a 6 again.

MERIDIANS

The meridian system is the concept in Traditional Chinese Medicine of a path through which the life-energy known as *qi* (or *chi*) flows. Any meridian in harmony tends to lead to health and well-being. A system in disharmony is believed to lead to illness and disease. There are 12 standard meridian pathways.

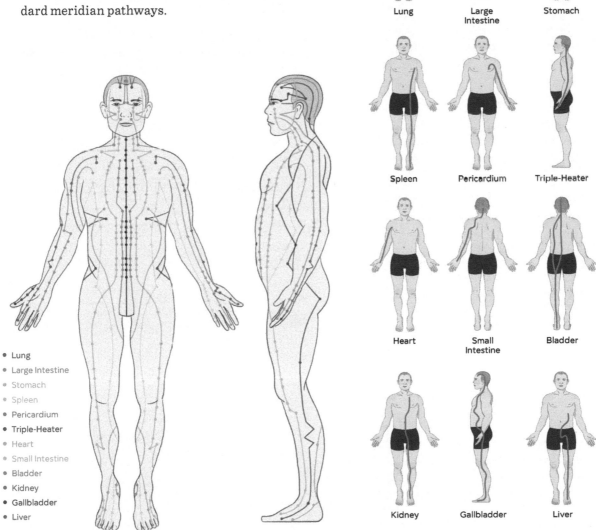

Lung

Large Intestine

Stomach

Spleen

Pericardium

Triple-Heater

Heart

Small Intestine

Bladder

Kidney

Gallbladder

Liver

- Lung
- Large Intestine
- Stomach
- Spleen
- Pericardium
- **Triple-Heater**
- Heart
- Small Intestine
- Bladder
- Kidney
- Gallbladder
- Liver

YIN & YANG

Yin and Yang are opposites in their individual qualities and nature, but they are also interdependent. Yin and Yang cannot exist without the other and they are constantly moving.

 Every single thing in our lives contains Yin and Yang—you can't have one without the other, and they are always in flux. So, when massaging the left side of the back, be sure to spend equal time on the other side for balance. This goes for other areas of the body as well, especially the feet, legs, hands, arms, and shoulders. Yin energy is believed to be night, lunar, feminine, and nurturing, while Yang is light, solar, masculine, and protecting.

There are 12 standard meridians, separated into Yin or Yang. For instance, the Yin meridians of the arm are the lung, heart, and pericardium. The Yang meridians of the arm are the large intestine, small intestine, and triple heater (see illustration on page 13).

CHAKRAS

The chakra system originated in India from an ancient text called the Vedas. The word "chakra" is derived from the Sanskrit word meaning "wheel." The seven chakras are the energy centers in our body through which energy flows. The essential chakras are stated in Buddhist and Hindu texts to be arranged in a column along the spinal cord, from its base to the top of the head, connected by vertical channels.

There are other minor chakras in the body, but here are the seven main ones:

1. **Root chakra (Muladhara)**
   Color: Red
   Location: Pelvis
   Spiritual purpose: Grounding, centering, balance.
   Physical purpose: The root chakra is associated with the gonadal (ovarian and testicular) systems, and and is believed to help balance sex hormones.

2. **Sacral chakra (Svadhisthana)**
   Color: Orange
   Location: Lower abdominal region
   Spiritual purpose: Well-being, pleasure, and creativity.
   Physical purpose: This chakra is associated with the adrenal glands and is believed to help regulate the immune system.

3. **Solar plexus chakra (Nabhi-Manipura)**
   Color: Yellow
   Location: Diaphragm
   Spiritual purpose: Confidence and self-esteem.
   Physical purpose: This chakra is associated with the pancreas and is believed to help regulate metabolism.

4. **Heart chakra (Anahata)**

   Color: Green

   Location: Center of the chest

   Spiritual purpose: Love and joy.

   Physical purpose: It is associated with the thymus gland and is believed to help regulate the immune system.

5. **Throat chakra (Vishuddhi)**

   Color: Blue

   Location: Throat

   Spiritual purpose: Communication and emotional expression.

   Physical purpose: It is associated with the thyroid gland and is believed to help regulate body temperature.

6. **Third eye chakra (Ana)**

   Color: Indigo

   Location: Between the eyebrows

   Spiritual purpose: Intuition, thinking, and making decisions.

   Physical purpose: This chakra is associated with the pituitary gland.

7. **Crown chakra (Sahasrara)**

   Color: Violet

   Location: Top of the head

   Spiritual purpose: Higher states of consciousness.

   Physical purpose: It is associated with the pineal gland and is believed to help regulate biological cycles.

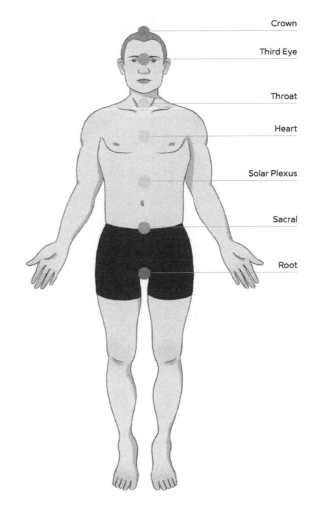

Crown

Third Eye

Throat

Heart

Solar Plexus

Sacral

Root

All of this should give you a foundation for understanding the body as a whole, complex machine with many interconnected systems. From the anatomy of the body to the anatomy of energy, this knowledge can support you as you learn to use massage in your life as a way to share the healing benefits with those around you or even yourself.

Putting It All Together

In this chapter, you've learned some of the basics of anatomy, the healing power of touch, and energy work. Now you're ready to learn some basic massage techniques. I hope you take the knowledge from this chapter with you through the rest of the book. The powerful mind-body connection is an important element of massage, no matter which style or technique you choose to work in.

In the upcoming chapters, I'll help you get started practicing massage and performing massage techniques for specific parts of the body, for certain types of pain, and specific types of people.

CHAPTER 2

Getting Started

Getting started with massage is easy—you really just need your hands. But there are a few considerations to keep in mind as you begin your journey with massage, such as creating a calm, inviting environment, maintaining a professional atmosphere (even when massaging friends or partners), and fully relaxing into the experience. You may also want to supplement your massages with oils, lotions, and music, or purchase a massage table or special linens. In this chapter, I outline everything you need to know to get started, including eight must-know massage techniques.

Giving & Receiving

The benefits of receiving massage are widely known, but massage therapists report experiencing meaningful benefits from giving massage as well. It is empowering to be able to give someone so much relief. I consider myself a caregiver, so I want to do everything in my power to help a person. The greatest feeling for me is when I'm finished and my client has a relaxed look on their face; this show of appreciation is so gratifying.

AN OFFERING

I teach my students that giving massages should always be professional, and performed without expectation. This is true even when giving your partner or a friend a massage. I encourage you to view massage as an intimate, healing act in its own right, and not in exchange for something. The exchange between massage practitioner and recipient is an offering that goes far beyond an exchange of money or anything else. It's a sacred act. For the receiver, it's about surrendering the body for healing and relaxation. For the giver, it's about offering your healing touch to another.

RELAXING & SURRENDER

Part of this offering is in showing up fully to your massage. Whether you're the giver or receiver, leave all your worries at the door when you enter for your massage. Getting yourself emotionally ready is vital to receiving the greatest benefits from massage.

As the receiver, start by visualizing yourself on the massage table and letting all your worries and to-dos melt into the table. As the giver, place your hands on the recipient for a few moments before beginning. This quiet moment of connection allows you both to get comfortable with touch and begin to relax into the experience. The best thing to do is to slowly ease into the massage. It should never begin with vigorous techniques. You can also have them take a few deep breaths to help induce the relaxation response. It's up to you as the giver to create this gentle transition into the massage.

A RELAXING ENVIRONMENT

A relaxing environment is an essential part of the massage experience. Whether you're giving a massage at home or in a professional setting, the atmosphere alone can encourage relaxation before you even begin the massage.

Here are a few recommendations for creating a soothing setting:

Music or white noise is great for creating a relaxing environment. The music you choose should be soothing with limited or no words. When I had my business, I always asked my clients what kind of music they would like. I've even given massages to heavy metal! That's why it's important to ask and not assume what is most relaxing for the client. For instance, I had one client who didn't want any music; I later found out that she was a music teacher and automatically analyzed music whenever she heard it, so it was not relaxing for her.

Aromatherapy can also be relaxing, but you need to make sure the recipient is okay with the scent and doesn't have allergies. There are a lot of essential oils to choose from such as lavender, mandarin, ginger, and more. I cover more essential oils in chapter six (page 150).

You also want to consider the temperature; ideally, the indoor temperature should be around 75 degrees Fahrenheit. The longer you massage someone, the more likely they are to get cold, especially in exposed areas not being massaged. I always cover the area with a sheet if I'm not massaging it.

Dim, soft lighting is more relaxing; very bright lights can be distracting and energizing. I like to keep the room dimly lit so that boundaries are clear and I can spot a bruise, lesion, rash or anything of concern I may need to ask the client about. The main thing is creating maximum comfort and relaxation for the recipient.

MASSAGE SUPPLIES

You can give a great massage at home without a table, but even many beginners eventually invest in some kind of table. Massage tables can range from a hundred dollars to thousands of dollars. Portable massage tables are an affordable option and there are many kinds to choose from, such as electric or hydraulic. No matter what, be sure to buy a table from a reputable company that offers a warranty.

If a massage table is not in your budget, you can use a bed. The biggest problem when using a bed is that you will have to reach over the recipient's body more. What I like to do when working on a bed is massage one side of the body, then ask the receiver to move to the other side of the bed, where I can start working on the other side of the body.

There's no need to spring for fancy massage linens. Usually these are just twin-size sheets anyway! When working at a table, you can use a pillowcase to put over the headrest. I prefer flannel sheets, because they are warmer. It's important to wash your sheets after every use and to always use a clean set of sheets for each new recipient. Don't forget to disinfect the table, too.

MASSAGE OILS & MORE

The good news is, you don't have to break the bank buying fancy massage supplies. For massage oils, you can simply use jojoba oil, or even extra-virgin olive oil that you may even use at home already or grape-seed oil. I personally prefer grape-seed oil, because it absorbs into the skin faster, leaving you less likely to slip. If you want to mix it up, professional grade massage oils are widely available at a reasonable price. Although, if you or anyone you plan on massaging has a history of allergic reactions, be sure to look for hypoallergenic oils.

In addition to oils, the other popular massage lubricants are, lotions, gels, and creams. These are also affordable and easy to find. I recommend trying them all and getting a sense of what works best for you and the varying needs of your massages. Here's what to know about each.

Massage oil is the most popular choice. It's excellent for gliding (page 24). Some people complain that they feel too greasy after a massage with oil, but this really depends on how much oil you use. It's always better to start the massage with a small amount of oil. You can always add more if needed. If you apply too much oil on the body, it takes a while to remove the excess, and your hands will probably slip too much. A general rule of thumb for a full body massage is about one to two ounces of massage oil. Two ounces if you perform a lot of gliding techniques, and one ounce or less if you don't.

Massage lotion is more water-based than regular lotion and it will also help you glide on the body. It's a great choice for people who don't want to feel oily after a massage, but it can be painful for massage recipients with hairy chests and backs. Keep in mind that massage lotion absorbs quicker than other lubricants, so you'll need to reapply more often.

Massage gel is a paraffin-based lubricant, and it stays on the body a lot longer than other lubricants.

I find that it's the best lubricant for people with more hair on their body, because it's less likely to entangle their hair. It also absorbs slowly, so you can perform more extended gliding techniques without needing to reapply.

Massage cream has also become popular in recent years. I find that it gives a great balance of absorption and glide. You don't have to apply it as much as massage lotion and recipients typically don't have that greasy feeling after a massage.

The Eight Must-Know Techniques to Get Started

While there are literally thousands of different massage techniques, they can usually be grouped into eight categories: effleurage (gliding), petrissage (kneading), friction, tapotement (percussion), vibration, feathering (light/stroking), compression, and stretching. These all stem from Swedish massage (page 71), which is arguably the best-known style in the West and the foundation for modern massage. Some therapists believe there are many more categories but having a strong understanding of these eight techniques is a great starting point. There are many variations of each, which you'll explore as you get more experience.

PRESSURE

One of the most common complaints from massage clients is the level of pressure—either the pressure is too deep, or too light. It is important to ask for feedback and encourage them to tell you if the pressure is ever too much. A little discomfort is okay, but when they start tensing up in response, that can defeat the whole purpose of the massage.

Gliding (Effleurage)

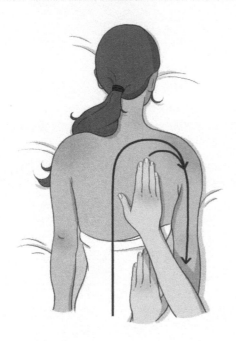

Effleurage, also known as gliding, is one of the most common techniques in massage. This technique is excellent for starting a massage and applying oil to the body before you perform deeper work.

1. Apply enough lubricant to your hands so you can perform this technique a few times in a row without needing to reapply.

2. Place both of your hands at their lower back.

3. Slowly glide up their back and then down their arm.

4. You can either slide both hands at the same time or alternate your hands.

5. Repeat 3–5 times on each side.

Kneading (Petrissage)

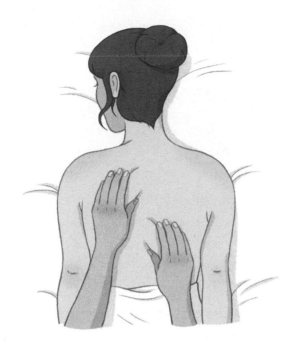

Petrissage, or kneading, is a technique that allows you to apply deeper pressure without pushing down on the recipient. This technique is used to lift the skin, muscles, and fascia. You don't need a lot of oil for this technique. If you have too much, it's harder to lift, hold onto, and manipulate the muscles.

1. Do not apply extra oil before you perform this technique.

2. Place both of your hands on the recipient's body.

3. Alternate lifting up the skin and softly grabbing muscles and fascia between your thumb and fingers.

4. Perform this technique 3–5 times in the same area.

5. After you're done with one area, go to another area and continue performing the technique.

Friction

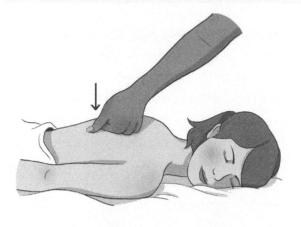

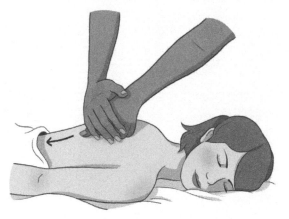

Friction is a broader massage technique. It should always be performed after you've warmed up an area using long, flowing motions for 1–2 minutes.

1. Starting at the shoulders of the recipient, make a fist with one of your hands, and extend your thumb.

2. Use your other hand to cover, support, and firmly press your thumb into the muscle.

3. Maintaining pressure, slowly glide your thumb either down the length of the muscle or against the muscle grain (this is known as cross-fiber friction).

4. Repeat this technique 3–5 times in the same area, increasing your pressure each time depending on what your recipient can tolerate.

Percussion (Tapotement)

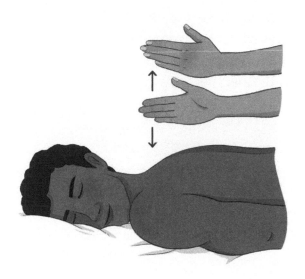

Tapotement, or percussion, is a commonly used technique. While it may not appear to be relaxing, the truth is that it *can* be quite relaxing if you start out lighter and gradually tap harder. This technique benefits all layers of the muscles.

1. No oil is used with this technique.

2. Make sure your hands and wrists are completely relaxed. You'll make a flicking motion with your hand.

3. With the pinky side of your relaxed hand, lightly strike the body in the desired area.

4. After a few times, you can increase the pressure depending on the recipient's tolerance and desire.

5. Repeat for 20–30 seconds, then move to another area.

Note: Do not perform this on any bony areas, pulse locations, or other endangerment sites.

Vibration

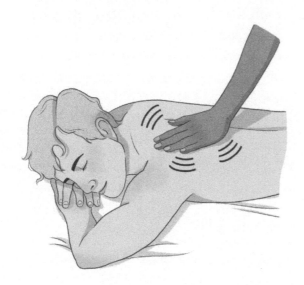

Vibration is a great technique to get a sense of how relaxed your massage recipient is. Try this technique after you've used other methods in an area.

1. Do not apply any extra oil.

2. Place your hand on the skin and slowly move your hand back and forth, keeping your hand and wrist relaxed.

3. Increase the pressure and speed of the vibration depending on your recipient's preferences.

4. Repeat for 10–20 seconds in each area.

Feathering

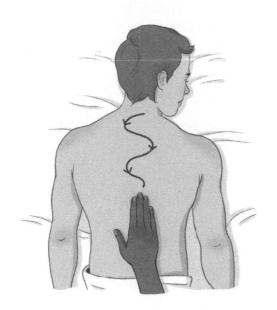

Feathering is a gentler technique that's generally used as you're getting started with a massage. You never want to start out with this method, because it can be ticklish for some people.

1. Do not add any extra oil for this technique.
2. Slowly glide your fingers or hands in a zigzag motion very lightly over the area.
3. Repeat 3–5 times.

Compression

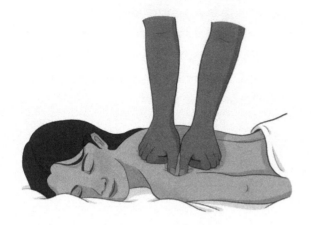

Compression should be performed after you've warmed up an area for 1–2 minutes with other methods. (Starting with this technique would be a big shock to the system.) Compression is the technique often used to access trigger points.

1. After you've warmed up an area, make a fist with both hands, and extend your thumbs (holding them tightly to your index fingers).

2. Slowly sink your thumbs into the muscles, applying firm pressure. Hold the pressure for 10–30 seconds.

3. After your recipient has relaxed, have them take a deep breath, and when they breathe out, slowly increase your pressure to the next layer of muscles.

4. Continue this technique 3–5 times on the area.

Stretching

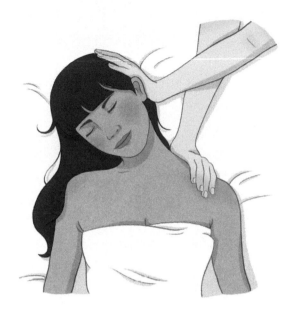

Stretching can be just as relaxing as pressure when performed right. You can also access areas on the body that are harder to reach in a massage.

1. Have your recipient take a few deep breaths.

2. Cross your hands and place one of your hands on their shoulder.

3. Place your other hand on the side of their head.

4. Slowly push your hands in opposite directions, until you feel a little resistance from the recipient.

5. Hold the stretch for 20–30 seconds.

6. After the 20–30 seconds, slowly bring their head back to a neutral position and take your hands off their head and shoulder.

7. Repeat 2–3 times if the recipient prefers more stretching. Then switch to the other side.

CHAPTER 3

Techniques for the Whole Body

People have different preferences about which body part to work on first in a massage. I prefer to begin with the face and scalp because I can do these areas before putting any oil on my hands. Others prefer to start massaging the back because that tends to be a common problem area, and that way you can finish with the recipient's face up, their sinuses drained. Wherever you choose to start, it's important to give yourself time guidelines so you can give enough attention to all the areas your recipient would like massaged. This chapter walks you through techniques for different body parts, starting with the head and face and working your way down for a full body massage.

Moving Through the Body

For a full body 60-minute massage, here's how I like to break it down.

Start by having the recipient lie face up. This is called the supine position, and allows you to work on the front part of the body, known as the anterior.

- 5 minutes: Face and scalp
- 5 minutes: Neck and shoulders
- 5 minutes: Right arm and hand
- 5 minutes: Left arm and hand
- 5 minutes: Right leg and foot
- 5 minutes: Left leg and foot

Now, ask them to flip over and lie face down (called the prone position). This is when you'll massage the backside of their body, known as the posterior.

- 5 minutes: Right leg and foot
- 5 minutes: Left leg and foot
- 20 minutes: Back, neck and shoulder

Of course, feel free to modify this general routine if someone needs more attention on a certain area, or if they don't want specific areas massaged. Be sure to explain how you'll be allocating the time if you devote a large chunk to one area. This way there will be no surprises at the end, like, "Hey, how come you never got to my feet?"

For a 30-minute massage, plan to target just the back, neck, or a specific problem area. It's difficult to give a full body massage in a half hour, unless you're working with a geriatric recipient, on children, or your recipient only wants a couple of minutes for each body part.

If you're at home and only have 10–15 minutes to give a massage (or your partner is begging you for a quick one), have them sit in a chair and massage their neck and shoulders. Or have them lie on a couch or on a bed and massage their feet.

In a professional setting, 90-minute massages have become more popular, which I'm glad about. These longer times give the massage therapist more time to focus on problem areas, while still providing a complete full body massage. It's the whole package. I've found that most people prefer to have more time devoted to their back, with neck and shoulders a close second.

The Head

Since this part of the body isn't touched by others as frequently as the hands or the arms, it's a good idea to gently place your hands on the scalp or face for a few seconds before you start massaging. This allows your recipient to get accustomed to your touch. I've always told my students that hair is an extension of the body and it needs a massage, too. If someone has a thicker head of hair, they can typically handle more vigorous scalp and hair techniques. Here are three of my favorite head techniques.

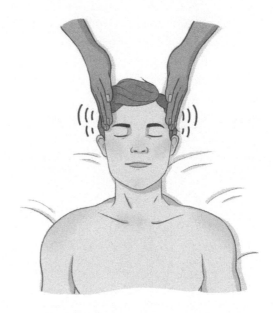

Temple Turn

1. Start with no oil on your hands.
2. Place your fingertips on their temple region.
3. Apply friction (page 26) in a circular motion.
4. Perform the technique 3–5 times.

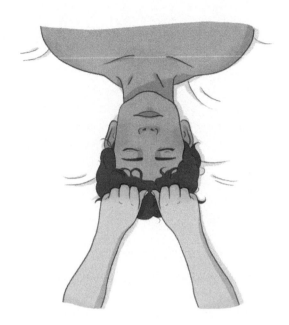

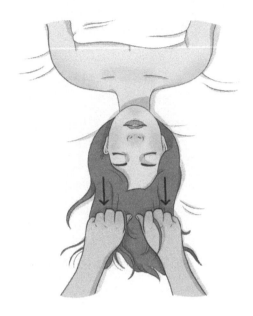

Skritchies

1. Start with no oil on your hands.
2. Use both of your hands to grasp some of their hair.
3. Lightly pull and hold for 5–10 seconds.
4. Perform the technique 3–5 times.

Slide & Hold

1. Start with no oil on your hands.
2. Place your hands on their scalp.
3. Slowly pull their hair while gliding (page 24) all the way to the tips of their hair.
4. Perform the technique 3–5 times.

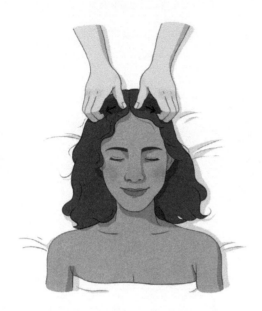

Hair Part

1. Start with no oil on your hands.
2. Place your hands on the top of their head.
3. Use your thumbs to part their hair.
4. Perform the technique 3–5 times.

INDIAN HEAD MASSAGE

Indian head massage is an ancient treatment that has been practiced in India for thousands of years. It is part of Ayurvedic medicine (also called Ayurveda, page 101), one of the world's oldest medical systems. Ayurveda is made up of the three doshas, or types of energy: *Vata* (air energy), *pitta* (fire energy), and *kapha* (water energy). These are dynamic forces of nature, and working principles that help us to understand our bodies better.

Here's a routine for a basic Indian head massage.

1. Have them sit in a chair fully clothed.
2. Place your hands on their shoulders without moving for a few seconds to get them used to your touch.
3. Start by slowly adding circular friction techniques (page 26) on their shoulders for 20–30 seconds with your thumbs.
4. Gently squeeze their shoulders with your hands and increase the pressure to what they can tolerate.
5. Place one of your hands on their forehead for support and place your other hand on the back of their neck. Slowly squeeze and use circular friction along the sides of their neck with your thumb and fingers.
6. Place both hands on top of their scalp and use circular friction techniques all around the scalp.

The Face

Face massage can be extremely relaxing and is one of the reasons many people get facials. If you choose to use lotion for massaging the face, make sure it's hypoallergenic, and that you get their permission to use it first. Many people have sensitive skin or are particular about the products they put on their face. I find you rarely need a lubricant for facial massage, as the skin on most people's faces is naturally supple and naturally oily.

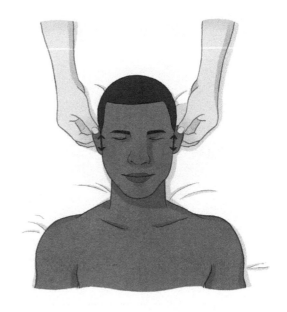

Ear Slide

1. Start with no oil on your hands.
2. Slowly apply friction (page 26) using a back and forth motion on the front and back of their ears, up and down their ears.
3. Either perform it one ear at a time, or both at the same time.
4. Perform the technique 3–5 times.

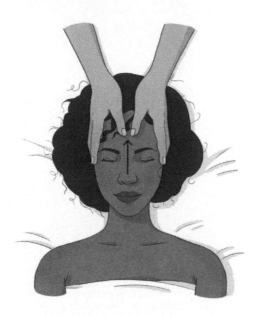

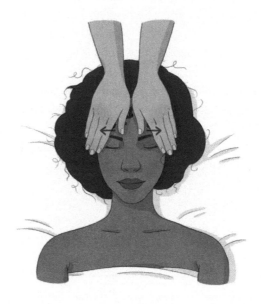

Third Eye Slide

1. Start with no oil on your hands.
2. Slowly glide (page 24) up the middle of your recipient's forehead, from the top of their nose to their hairline.
3. You can create friction back and forth.
4. Perform the technique 3–5 times.

Forehead Split

1. Start with no oil on your hands.
2. Place your thumbs or fingers at the center of their forehead.
3. Slowly glide (page 24) your hands apart, ending close to their ears.
4. Perform the technique 3–5 times.

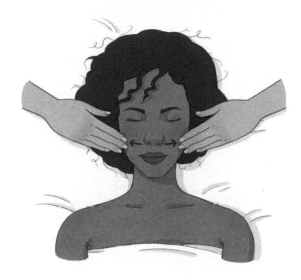

Sinus Drain

1. Start with no oil on your hands.

2. Place your fingertips close to their nose, under their cheekbones.

3. Slowly glide (page 24) under their cheekbones, away from their nose, up toward their ears.

4. Perform the technique 3–5 times.

The Neck

The neck is a vital part of any massage. In today's tech age, with so many hours spent hunched over screens and mobile devices, many people suffer from neck and shoulder pain. Additionally, many headaches start in the neck and shoulders, and one of the most significant problem spots is right under the base of the skull. You can use oil on the neck—I recommend it—but be mindful not to get oil in the hair or face.

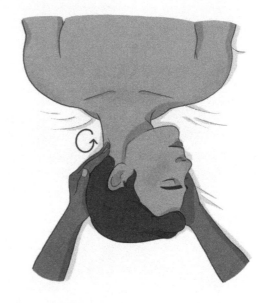

Turn & Dig

1. Add oil to your hands. Start this technique with a supporting hand under their head (if you're worried about getting oil in their hair, use a towel or pillowcase as a barrier).

2. Slowly turn their head.

3. Find the base of the skull, and slowly glide (page 24) under it, or hold pressure on a tender area (bring the discomfort to 6–7 out of 10) until the pain dissipates.

4. If you're using a gliding technique with your fingertips, repeat the technique 3–5 times, and increase the pressure a little more each time.

5. After you've finished on that side, slowly turn their head to the other side and repeat.

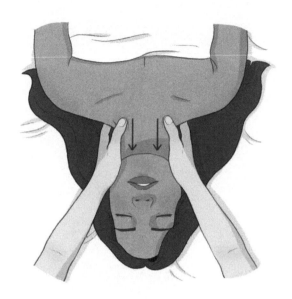

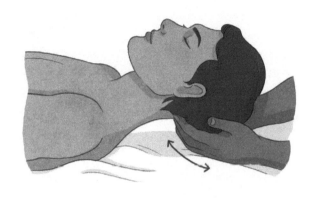

Long Neck

1. Add oil to your hands,

2. Place your hands on their shoulders.

3. Slowly glide (page 24) up their neck with both hands.

4. To modify, alternate gliding your hands up their neck. This will help you isolate one side at a time.

5. Perform the technique 3–5 times.

Skull Rock

1. Have little to no oil on your hands.

2. With both hands, lift their head off the table or surface, and place your fingertips under the base of their skull.

3. Slowly rock their head up and down (the direction from their head to their feet).

4. You don't need to add any extra pressure, because the weight of their head will do that.

5. Continue this technique for 10–20 seconds. Repeat 3–5 times.

The Shoulders

One of the more significant problems with shoulders is that people tend to hunch them for most of the day, keeping them internally rotated. Or they have "shoulder rings" (one of my students coined that phrase for people who elevate their shoulders too much). Having your body in an unnatural position at work for a long period of time can cause undue stress on your shoulder muscles and make them tight. These techniques may help with that.

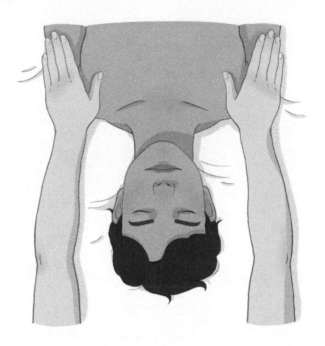

Hold Me Down

1. Place your hands on the anterior part of their shoulders.
2. Slowly push the shoulders down toward the table and hold for 5–10 seconds until the recipient feels a little pressure.
3. Perform the technique 3–5 times.

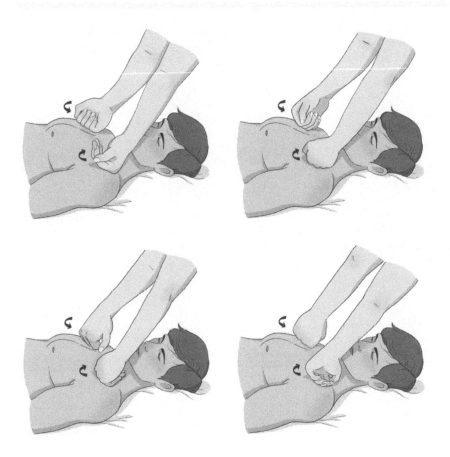

Grind Pecs

1. Add a little oil to your knuckles.
2. Place your knuckles in their upper pectoral region (see Muscular System, page 10).
3. Slowly turn your knuckles in a circular motion.
4. Increase the pressure as the recipient desires.
5. Perform the technique 3–5 times.

The Back

The back is the core part of your massage. Almost everyone wants the most time spent in this area. The back, back of the neck, shoulders, mid back, and lower back are usually included in a back massage. Since there are a few layers of muscles in the back, it is crucial to warm up the muscles. Be sure to start slowly and gradually increase pressure—if you use too much pressure to start, the body tends to tense up, and it becomes harder for the recipient to relax. Be mindful of the antagonist/opposite muscles, which we address in the abdominal section (page 52).

One big complaint when massaging the back is too much oil. It's tempting to slather it on with such a large area, but it's always better to use a little less to start with because you can always add more. If you add too much, you are more than likely to slip on a muscle or into the spine when performing more in-depth work. I usually start at the shoulders and use extended techniques gliding down to their lower back so that I can apply oil to the whole back slowly throughout the process.

For these techniques, your recipient should be face down (in prone position).

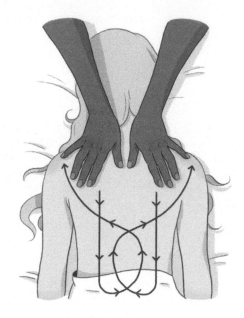

Figure 8

1. Stand on one side of the table near their head or shoulder.
2. Place your hands on their shoulders.
3. Glide (page 24) both your hands down to their lower back.
4. Stop briefly at their lower back, or just continue the flow of the technique.
5. Glide your hands back to their shoulders crossing your hands as you come back up, tracing a figure 8 shape.
6. Perform the technique 3–5 times.

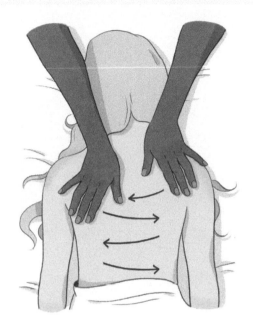

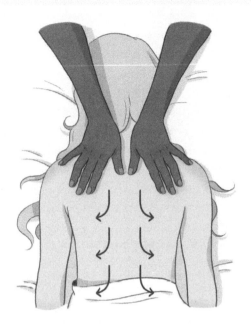

Full Fan

1. Stand on one side of the table near their head or shoulder.

2. Glide (page 24) one hand down both sides of the back.

3. Alternate your hands doing this motion, working your way down their body.

4. After you have reached their lower back, bring your hands back to their shoulders, either by gliding back to the starting point or lifting your hands off the lower back and carry them back to the shoulders.

5. Perform the technique 3–5 times.

Half Fan

1. Stand on one side of the table near their head or shoulder.

2. Place your hands on their shoulders.

3. Glide (page 24) your hands down to their lower back with both hands, using short strokes in opposite directions.

4. Perform the technique 3–5 times.

The Arms

Massaging the arms is also great for people with desk jobs. In a full body massage, the back of the arms (triceps region) often gets neglected. To avoid this, massage the triceps when they are face down while you're massaging their back. Be careful to not use too much pressure on the biceps region because that area is more prone to bruising. If someone has very thin arms, use your fingertips more. If the arm is hairy, avoid lotion because it will dry and pull the hair. Oil is the best option.

I always massage one arm and then the hand on the same side, and then move to the other arm and hand.

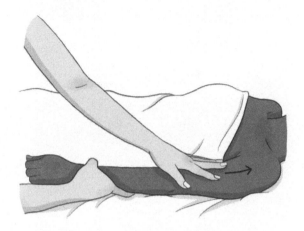

Traction Glide

1. Place one of your hands on their wrist.

2. Add a little oil on your other hand.

3. Gently pull their wrist with your supporting hand and use the other hand to glide (page 24) up their arm to their shoulder.

4. Perform the technique 3–5 times.

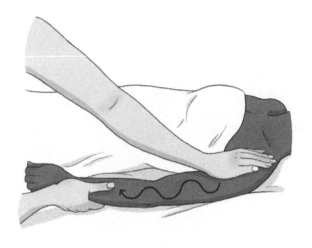

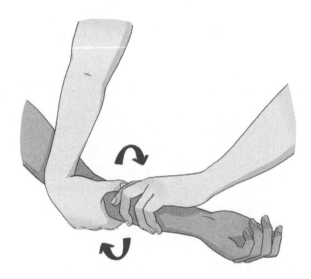

Wiggle Arm

1. Do not add any extra oil.
2. Place one of your hands on their wrist to add support. Start with the other hand on their shoulder.
3. Gently wiggle their arm with your fingers from their shoulder to wrist.
4. Perform the technique 3–5 times.

Snake Bite

1. Don't add any extra oil.
2. Place your hands and fingers around their forearm.
3. Slowly twist your hands in opposite directions to the point of a little discomfort.
4. Hold for 2–5 seconds.
5. Perform the technique 3–5 times.

The Hands

Most of us use our hands a lot for our jobs, and it can be beneficial to anyone to receive a hand massage. Research shows that massage is an effective treatment for carpal tunnel syndrome. You can either use oil or lotion, but if you do use oil, it is a good idea to remove the oil with a towel after you're done. Be sure to give the back of the hand as much attention as the palm, because they are the antagonist (opposite) to each other.

It is possible to massage one of your hands with your other hand, but it is a lot easier (and more relaxing) to have someone else perform it.

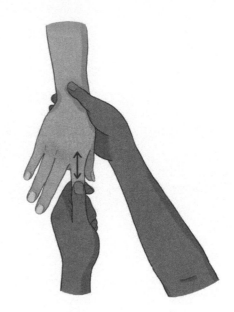

Finger Pulling

1. Add a little oil to your hands.
2. Use one hand to support their wrist.
3. Lift up their wrist with your supporting hand.
4. Use your other hand to friction (page 26) off each finger.
5. Repeat on each finger and the thumb 3–5 times.

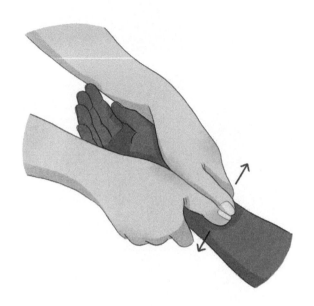

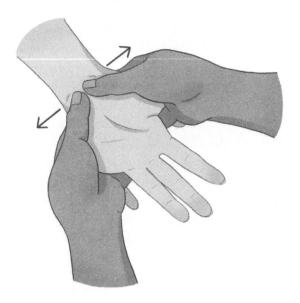

Wrist Spread

1. Add a little oil to your hands.
2. Wrap your fingers around their wrist. Place your thumbs in the center of their wrist.
3. Slowly slide your thumbs in opposite directions toward the outsides of the wrist.
4. Perform the technique 3–5 times.

Pinky, Pinky, Wrap It, Spread It

1. Lift one hand with their palm facing up.
2. Interlock one of your pinkies between their ring and pinky finger, and your other pinky between their thumb and index fingers.
3. Wrap your fingers around their hand.
4. Place your thumbs at the base of their palm.
5. Slowly spread their palm with your thumbs.
6. Keep your hands in the same position and glide your thumbs around their palm in different directions or just use one thumb at a time to isolate an area.
7. Repeat 3–4 in different areas on their palm.

The Stomach

The abdominal area is often skipped in a massage treatment—either the giver doesn't feel confident massaging that area, or the recipient doesn't want it for various reasons. However, I'm a strong believer in including it because most of the abdominal muscles are the antagonist (opposite actions) of the back muscles. When one muscle is weak or injured, then the antagonist muscle will have to do more work. It is important not to push straight down on the abdominal muscles, and massage at an angle to the receiver's comfort level. Always check with the recipient before massaging this area.

The receiver should be on their back for these techniques. While most men feel comfortable with their chest exposed, be sure to cover women recipients when using this technique.

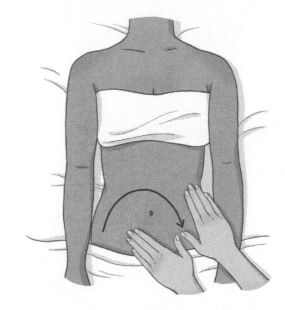

Lower Stomach Rub

1. Add some oil to your hands.
2. Stand on the left side of their body.
3. Place your hands on their lower colon region (just above the right hip).
4. Slowly glide (page 24) your hands in the direction of the colon (gliding straight up from the right hip to the lower ribs, then straight across, and finally gliding down from their lower left ribs to their left hip). You can do this with your hands together, or alternate hands with your gliding.
5. Perform the technique 3–5 times.

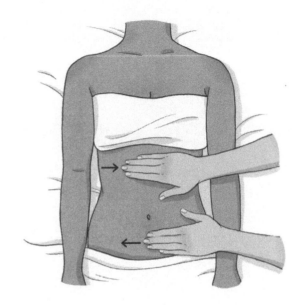

Colon Burn

1. Add some oil to your hands.

2. Stand on the left or right side of their body and place your hands on the opposite side of the body, halfway between their hip and lower ribs.

3. Alternate your hands going back and forth in a light and fast wave-like motion.

4. Perform this technique 20–30 seconds.

The Glutes (Buttocks)

The buttocks, or the glute region, is made up of three main muscles: the gluteus maximus, gluteus medius, and the gluteus minimus. Massaging the glutes is beneficial because the muscles of the glutes can refer pain to the lower back. It is a good idea to warm up each muscle layer of the glutes before applying a lot of pressure to the area. Using your knuckles and elbows is a great way to increase pressure for people who like deeper work. Never add pressure to the ball and socket region of the hip (known as the greater trochanter); it can cause bruising.

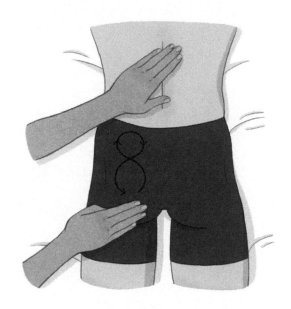

Figure 8 Glutes

1. Add a little oil to one of your knuckles.
2. Place one hand on their lower back for support.
3. Glide (page 24) your knuckles in figure 8 motions around one side of the glutes (make sure you don't add pressure to the ball and socket of the hip).
4. Perform the technique 3–5 times.

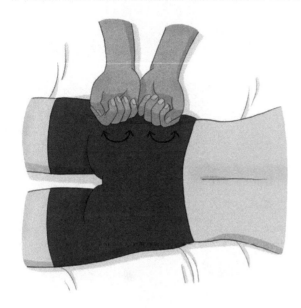

Knuckle Glutes

1. Add a little oil to the knuckles of both hands.

2. Place both hands on their glutes.

3. Glide (page 24) in figure 8 motions around the glute. Make sure you don't add pressure to their great trochanter (the ball and socket of the hip).

4. Perform the technique 3–5 times.

The Thighs

The thighs can be a sensitive area to massage, especially the inner region. Be sure to drape the groin region properly, so nothing is exposed. The hamstring and quad muscles are antagonist to each other, so be sure to give adequate attention to both sides of this region.

If the receiver has problems with their knees, massaging the thighs can be beneficial because those muscles all connect to the knee area. Research has also shown that massage may help with pain due to osteoarthritis of the knee. Oil is preferable for this area of the body, as lotion may cause uncomfortable friction when it dries on hair.

When massaging the quads, have the recipient lie face up (supine), and for massaging hamstrings, have them face down (prone).

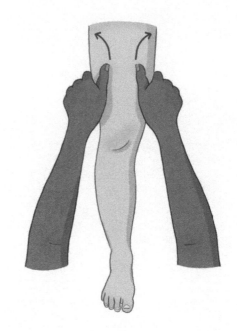

Squash

1. Add oil to your hands.
2. Place your hands on the center of their thigh, halfway between the hip and the knee.
3. Slowly separate your hands (one hand going to the outer thigh and the other hand going to the inner thigh).
4. You can perform this technique on the hamstrings, too (when the recipient is face down).
5. Perform this technique 3–5 times, increasing the pressure a little more each time.

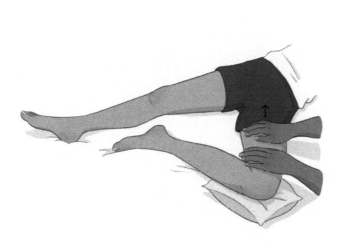

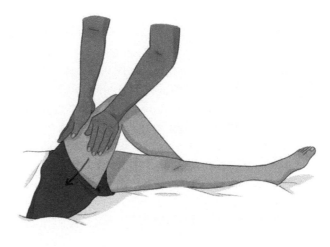

Make a Wish

1. Bend one knee and rotate it outwards.
2. If they lack flexibility, place a pillow or bolster under their knee.
3. Massage the inside of their thigh with slow circular motions, kneading (page 25), or gliding (page 24).
4. Massage for 20–30 seconds using different techniques.

Cross Over Slide

1. Bend one of their knees and place their foot over their bottom leg.
2. Place one of your hands on their knee and press down to give the lateral thigh a good stretch.
3. Slowly glide (page 24) up and down the outer thigh with your forearm or palm for 20–30 seconds.

The Calves

Calves are a great place to concentrate for people who work on their feet all day, but there are some precautions to be aware of. Older people, those who are pregnant, and long-haul travelers are more prone to having DVT (deep vein thrombosis), a potentially deadly type of blood clot that forms in the calves. Make sure you are aware of the signs and symptoms of DVT. If they have intense pain, swelling, and tenderness in their calf, it's best not to massage the area, and you may wish to advise your client to contact a medical professional. If there is no risk of DVT, give equal attention to both the front (anterior) and back (posterior) of the lower legs.

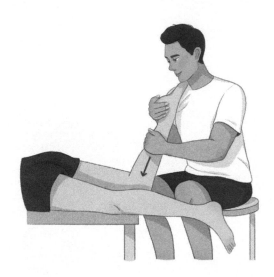

Shoulder Support

1. With the recipient face down in the prone position, lift one foot, bending their knee.

2. Apply oil to one or both of your hands. You can place a towel on your shoulder to protect your clothes from the oil.

3. Use one hand to support their ankle and hold it in place.

4. With your other hand, glide (page 24) up and down their calf region with superficial gliding techniques first, increasing the pressure a little more each time. You will only massage the calf region.

5. Perform the technique 3–5 times, and then alternate your hands.

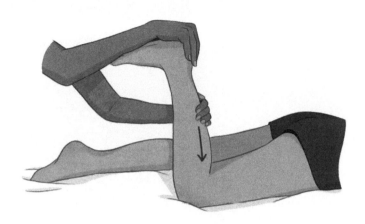

Dorsi Slide

1. Have the recipient lie face down (prone position).

2. Add a little oil to your hands.

3. Lift up their foot.

4. Cup their heel with one hand and stretch out their calf with your forearm to the recipient's desired stretch.

5. Glide down their calve with your other hand, increasing the pressure a little each time.

6. Perform the technique 3–5 times.

The Feet

People either love or hate to have their feet massaged. When people say they don't like their feet massaged, it's usually because they are ticklish. Luckily, I've found an almost fool-proof way to work around sensitive feet: Place a towel or sheet over their feet and massage 30–60 seconds, remove the cloth and hold their feet for 5–10 seconds while adding pressure, and finally start massaging them making sure you use firm pressure. This generally helps mitigate the tickling sensation.

The benefits of foot massage are many, and according to Harvard Medical School, foot massage can improve circulation, stimulate muscles, reduce tension and ease pain.

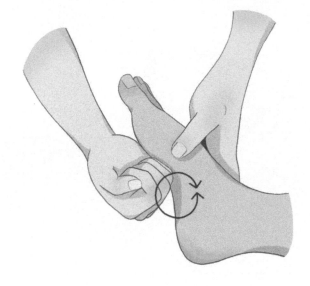

Knuckle Twist

1. Stand on one side of the table near the recipient's feet.
2. Place one of your hands on top of their foot to stabilize it.
3. Make a fist with your other hand.
4. Use your knuckles on the bottom of the foot, either using a gliding motion (page 24) or in a circular motion.
5. Continue with the technique for 20–30 seconds and add a little more pressure every 5–10 seconds.

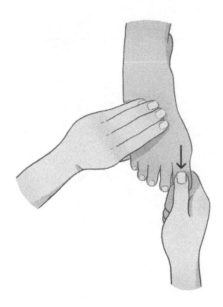

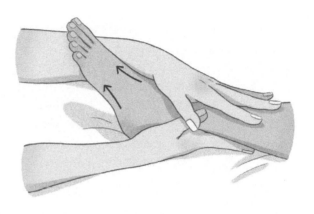

Slide Off Toe

1. Stand in front of their feet.

2. Place one of your hands on top of their foot to stabilize it.

3. Start at either the big or little toe and place your thumb and index finger at the base of the toe.

4. Slowly glide (page 24) off each toe, or you can use a pinching motion by fractioning off each toe.

5. After you have completed each toe, go back and perform the technique again 3–5 times on that foot.

Comfort Glide

1. Stand in front of their feet.

2. Place one of your hands on top of their ankle and the other one under their ankle.

3. Slowly slide your hands off their foot.

4. Repeat the technique 3–5 times, increasing the pressure to your recipient's comfort level.

Self-Massage

Self-massage can be challenging, especially on hard-to-reach areas. While it will never be as thorough as a partner massage, it's wonderful to know how to give yourself a massage for times of pain, or when you need to relax. Luckily you can use objects to help you "cheat" and reach some of those more hidden spots. Some of my favorite go-to tools: racquetball racquet, glass soda bottle (for the bottom of your foot), rolling pin, and tennis ball. When using a tool, be sure to start out with lighter pressure and slowly increase depending on how it feels.

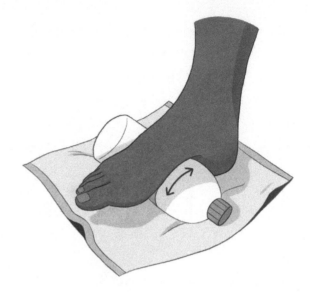

Plantar Self-Massage

1. For this technique, you can use a frozen water bottle, a racket ball, or rolling pin. Place the prop on carpet or a towel, so it doesn't slip.

2. Sit down if you don't have the right balance, or stand holding onto something for support.

3. Place the arch of your foot on the bottle and slowly roll the bottle back and forth, increasing the pressure a little more each time.

4. Continue this technique for 30–60 seconds.

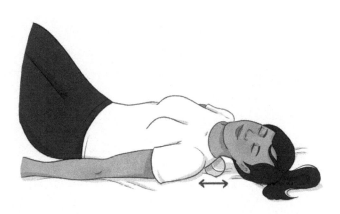

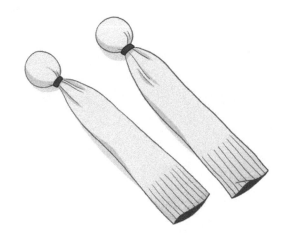

Tennis Ball

1. Lie on a nonslip floor or carpet, so the tennis ball doesn't slip.

2. Place the tennis ball on an area of discomfort. You can use the tennis ball technique on many areas of the body, including the back, back of the neck, arms, legs, and calves.

3. Slowly roll around in the area with the weight of your body.

4. Continue the technique 30–60 seconds, increasing the pressure a little more each time.

5. Do not place the ball under a bony area.

6. When you're finished, go to another area of the body.

Tennis Ball in a Sock

1. Place a tennis ball or racket ball in a sock.

2. Use a rubber band or ponytail holder to hold the ball at the end.

3. Either lie on your back on the floor or place your back against a wall.

4. Place the ball on a tender area on your back and hold on to the end of the sock.

5. Slowly move the sock around to different areas of your back.

6. Once you find a tender area, slowly roll around on that spot by having the weight of your body slowly increase the pressure by leaning into the ball.

CHAPTER 4

Techniques from Around the World

n this chapter, you'll learn sequences from some of the most effective and therapeutic massage styles from around the world that you can start incorporating into your practice. Having a basic understanding of these different massage modalities will help you discover the style that works best for you. If a certain style doesn't feel right, that's okay—try something else instead. Or combine them all! It's really a matter of preference. I tend to customize my massage techniques to what the client wants and not what I want for my clients. It's important to listen to what they say and then act on it. Here's a brief introduction to the different styles of massage.

Shiatsu

Shiatsu is a Japanese healing treatment based on the ideas of Traditional Chinese Medicine. Shiatsu means "finger pressure," and as such uses uses thumbs, fingers, elbows, and knees to access meridians (page 13). For this style of massage, the recipient is usually clothed and lying on a low massage table or comfortable pad on the floor. A more specific version of Shiatsu is acupressure, which is used to isolate certain pressure points to alleviate pain and dysfunction in the body. Shiatsu is more of a full body treatment that involves applying pressure to affect change in the body.

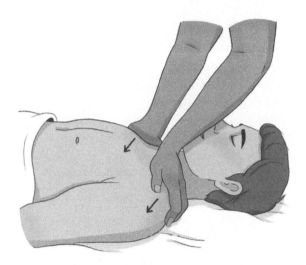

Rocking the Shoulders Technique

Using a side-by-side rocking technique relaxes the shoulders, and helps you feel which shoulder has less range of motion.

1. Start with your recipient face up (supine).
2. Place your hands on the front of their shoulders with your palms pressing into their shoulders.
3. Rock your hands back and forth, adding a little more pressure each time.
4. Continue for 20–30 seconds.

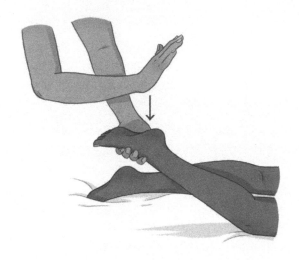

Hacking

This technique is good for accessing all the layers of the muscles. The areas where you can use this technique are: between the shoulder blades, mid back (never on the spine), hamstrings, quads, calves, biceps, and triceps. It's import to start out very light with this technique, and slowly add more speed, depth, and pressure to the receiver's comfort level.

1. Use only the heel of your hand.
2. Strike the body, slowly increasing the speed and depth to the person's desire.
3. Do not perform on bony areas, over organs, or on pulse regions.
4. Continue for 20–30 seconds in one area, then move to another one.

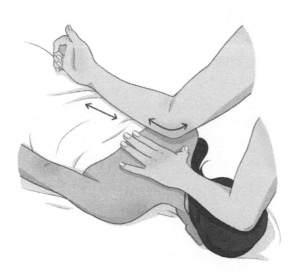

Elbow Rock

Using this technique can lessen the pressure more quickly than many other techniques, because you are not using stationary pressure. Each time you rock, you can increase the pressure a little more, encouraging the muscles to release. This technique can be used on other areas of the back, but never on the shoulder blades or spine.

1. Have the recipient lie face down (prone).
2. Place your elbow on their back (never on their spine).
3. Move your elbow up and down while slowly sliding down their back (like a jackhammer).
4. Increase the pressure each time, to the person's desire.
5. Repeat 3–5 times in one area, then move to another.

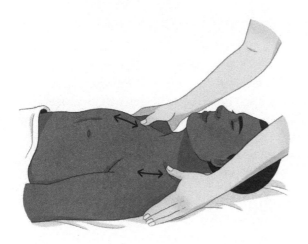

Rocking Your Thumbs

This technique can be used on the shoulders, but is also good for other areas of the body, especially along the sides of the spine.

1. Place your hands on opposite sides of an area of their body.

2. Rhythmically pump your thumbs up and down at the same time into that specific area of the body.

3. Increase the pressure to the person's comfort level.

4. Repeat 3–5 times in each area.

Swedish

Pehr Henrik Ling is credited with the development of modern Swedish massage, introducing it into the United States in 1858 as "The Swedish Movement Cure." It is a combination of gymnastics and physiology, pulled from Chinese, Egyptian, Greek, and Roman techniques. Swedish massage is the most common and best-known type of massage in the West, and is the foundation of other popular Western-style massages. It is typically the first style taught in massage schools, and a great foundation to start with to build on other styles. The Dutch practitioner Johan Georg Mezger is credited as the person who adopted the French names for the basic strokes of this style. Today it is known as "Swedish massage" in North America, and "classic massage" in Sweden.

With Swedish massage, the therapist uses massage oil and performs various massage techniques, including the primary methods for a traditional Swedish massage: effleurage, petrissage, friction, tapotement, vibration, nerve, and stretching (see The Eight Must-Know Techniques to Get Started, page 23, for more detail on these techniques).

ROLLER COASTER EFFECT

Swedish massage incorporates a roller coaster effect, meaning techniques can be slow, fast, or sporadic. Typically, the technique starts slow and light, then incorporates deeper pressure and some fast or rhythmic techniques, and finally ends with more relaxing and soothing techniques.

For example, use long flowing slow gliding techniques (page 24) to start, then move into fast gliding techniques once the area of their body is starting to relax. After that, slow it down with kneading techniques (page 25), followed by slower friction techniques (page 26). I usually finish an area of the body with feathering techniques (page 29).

Usually the techniques are performed 3–5 times each, to gradually induce a relaxation response in the body.

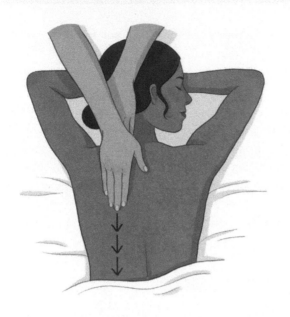

Shingles

This technique is great to use early on in a massage to spread oil onto the body. It is called shingles, because your hands overlap each other while you glide up, just as shingles are overlapped on a roof. Once you perform this on one side of the body perform it on the opposite side.

1. Add extra oil to your hands.
2. Have your recipient lie face down on the table (prone). Position your body on one the side of the table.
3. Place one hand over your other hand.
4. Slowly glide (page 24) up and pull up your bottom hand.
5. Place that hand over the other hand, while continuing the gliding motion.
6. Slowly glide up and pull out the bottom hand, placing it over the other hand.
7. Repeat this technique, gliding up and alternating hands, inching your way up their back.
8. Repeat the whole sequence 3–5 times.

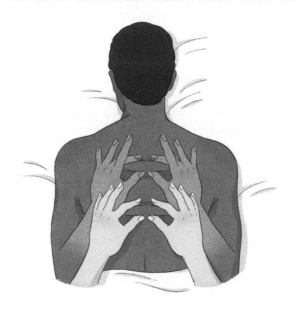

Skin Rolling

This technique is used to feel for restrictions in the fascia, muscles, and skin. When you feel a restriction, then you know that is a great place to focus more energy and techniques to help loosen it up. This technique is easiest to perform on the back, but can be used on other areas of the body if you can grasp the skin.

1. Use minimal oil on the area.
2. Point your thumbs together and place your hands on their back.
3. Lift up some skin and muscles with your index fingers while gliding your thumbs behind them.
4. Now use your middle fingers to lift up the skin and muscles while sliding your thumbs behind them.
5. Keep alternating your index and middle finger while gliding your thumbs. When you feel a restriction, you can stop and keep working in that isolated area before moving on to another area.

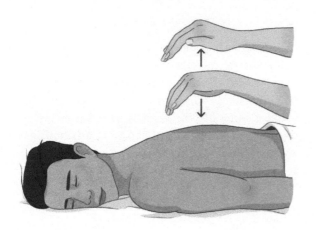

Cupping

Cupping can be used on the side of the ribs (upper side and back) to help break up phlegm. It sounds like a horse walking on a paved road, and you can increase the pressure and speed to the level they can handle.

1. No extra oil is needed for this technique.
2. Cup both of your palms and, with your wrists relaxed, alternate striking the body using percussion (page 27).
3. Stay away from any bony, pulse, or organ areas.
4. Continue this for 20–30 seconds.

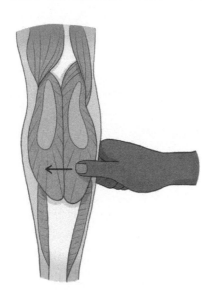

Cross My Fibers

This technique is great for resolving tightness or restrictions in the muscle and fascia.

1. Use a minimal amount of oil on the area.

2. Find the direction of the muscle being treated.

3. Slowly glide (page 24) across the muscle with your thumb.

4. Perform the method 3–5 times, and increase the pressure a little more each time.

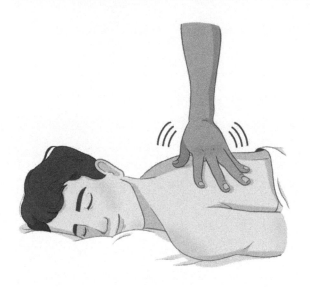

Fine Vibe

This technique might not seem relaxing at first, but the longer you perform it with rhythmic motions, the more you will feel the body relax.

1. Do not use any extra oil.
2. Extend your fingers and thumbs and place them on the body (as if you were performing a fingertip pushup).
3. Vibrate (page 28) your fingers and thumb back and forth for 10–20 seconds.
4. Vibrate other areas of the body if needed.

Deep Tissue

Deep tissue massage uses specific techniques to target problematic areas. It focuses on the deeper layers of muscles, tendons, and fascia as well as the superficial layers where dysfunction may also be causing pain. Deep Tissue is actually an umbrella term for trigger point therapy, neuromuscular therapy, myofascial release, and therapeutic massage.

Most people think deep tissue massage should cause discomfort, but that's not true. Many recipients are looking for a relieving kind of discomfort rather than a painful discomfort. Remember that the more a person tenses up during a deeper massage, the more likely they will be sore the next few days. It's essential and ethical to have open communication throughout this treatment; make sure they feel they can speak up, and make sure you're listening—ease up if it's ever too much pressure for your recipient.

With deep tissue massage, you'll be isolating a muscle or muscle group. It is best to warm up and relax the area with long flowing gliding techniques (page 24) or kneading (page 25) anytime you decide to use deep tissue in a specific area. Use minimal oil for deep tissue and you will be less likely to slip.

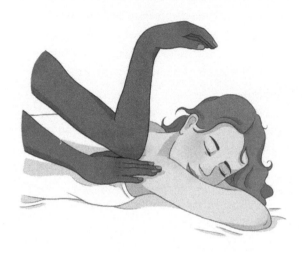

Elbow Ouch

This technique is used when you are not able to get enough pressure using your hands or fore-arms. Keep in mind that you have less sensation in your elbow, so make sure you communicate with your recipient to see if the pressure is okay and not too deep.

1. Make sure the muscles are warmed up before you use this technique.

2. Use a minimal amount of oil.

3. Cup your left elbow with your right hand to minimize slipping.

4. Find a tender muscle area on the body.

5. Slowly glide (page 24) over that area with your elbow, while supporting it with your other hand. You can also just stay in one place and let the pain dissipate as you press down with your elbow. This usually takes 10–15 seconds.

6. Perform 3–5 times, increasing the pressure a little more each time you slowly glide with your elbow.

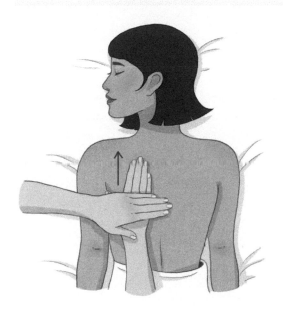

Hand Cross

This technique is great for adding extra pressure to an area where you would otherwise have problems adding enough pressure with one hand or your fingers. This technique is better for larger areas.

1. Make sure the muscles are warmed up before you use this technique.
2. Use a minimal amount of oil.
3. Find a tender muscle area on the body (the back is a great place to start).
4. Place one hand over your other hand for support.
5. Slowly glide (page 24) over that area, while supporting it with your other hand. The bottom hand is the one that glides, and your top hand is the one that adds pressure to the gliding hand.
6. Perform 3–5 times, increasing the pressure a little each time.

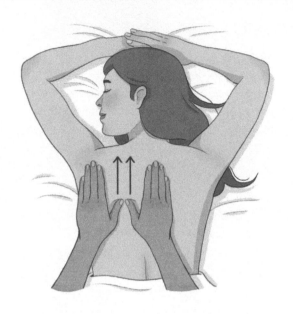

Two Thumb Slide

Thumbs are the best body part to use to feel for a difference (like a trigger point) in the muscle tissue. By sliding and pushing with your thumbs together, the thumbs have more support as they work.

1. Make sure the muscles are warmed up before you use this technique.

2. Use a minimal amount of oil.

3. Find a tender muscle area on the body.

4. Make a W with your thumbs.

5. Slowly glide (page 24) over that area, while pushing your thumbs into each other for support. The main pressure should come from your thumbs rather than the knuckles. Avoid the spine, bony areas, organ areas, and any place you can feel a pulse.

6. Perform 3–5 times, increasing the pressure a little each time.

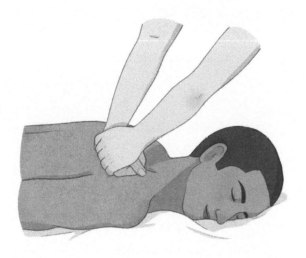

Hold My Thumb

This technique is great for increasing pressure and depth, while providing more support for your thumb.

1. Make sure the muscles are warmed up before you use this technique.
2. Make a fist and place your thumb over your index finger.
3. Place your other hand over your thumb for support.
4. Slowly glide (page 24) over the area.
5. Perform 3–5 times, increasing the pressure a little each time.

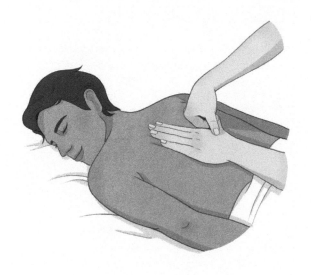

Knuckle Power

Supporting your knuckles will help you apply deep pressure without slipping.

1. Make sure the muscles are warmed up before you use this technique.

2. Use a minimal amount of oil.

3. Find a tender muscle area on the body.

4. Make an L on the area with one hand.

5. Place the knuckles of your other hand inside that L (the L hand is used as support).

6. Slowly glide (page 24) over that area with your knuckles.

7. Perform 3–5 times, increasing the pressure a little each time.

Sports Massage

Sports massage can be traced back thousands of years to Greece and Rome. In fact, the famous Roman physician Galen prescribed massage for athletes before and after exercising to help prevent injury and alleviate pain.

Modern sports massage can be documented in the 1924 Olympic games. Paavo Nurmi of Finland won five gold medals in the Olympic running competition, and he gave credit for his wins to the massages that he received from his massage therapist.

There are three types of sports massage (some say more, and others say less):

1. **Pre-event:** More invigorating massage techniques. These can be performed up to 24 hours before an event or just a few hours before. The purpose is to warm up the muscles.

2. **Post-event:** Typically more relaxing massage techniques and stretching. This can happen right after a game or hours after, and helps relax the athlete's muscles and mind.

3. **Maintenance:** Performed when an athlete has a reduced training schedule, is not competing, or during the athlete's off season, this massage targets problem areas before they become a bigger problem for peak performance time.

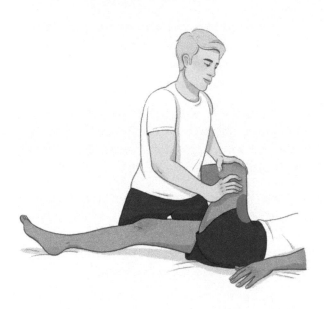

Intense TFL

The tensor fasciae latae (TFL) is the muscle that connects into the iliotibial band, the longest tendon in the body. To locate the TFL, find the hipbone and the outer side of the knee; the TFL is a tight band alongside the upper leg. It's a common muscle to target with sports massage and stretching, especially on athletes who use their legs a lot.

1. The recipient is on their back (supine).
2. Add a little oil to your hand that will be massaging.
3. Flex one of their knees. Stand on the side of the table opposite their bent knee.
4. Cross the bent leg over their bottom leg.
5. Rest the calf of the bent leg on the top of your hip.
6. Stretch out their TFL and glute region while holding their knee with your supporting hand.
7. Slowly glide on their hamstrings, quads, and TFL. It is best to use your palm to glide, and once it's warmed up, then you can increase the pressure using your knuckle or forearm.
8. Repeat 3–5 times, increasing the pressure each time.

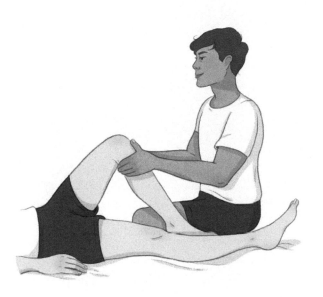

The Calf Spreader

This technique will help separate the superficial calf muscle (gastrocnemius), so you can access the deep calf muscle (soleus).

1. The recipient is on their back (supine).
2. Bend one of their knees.
3. Place that foot flat on the table.
4. Ask permission to sit on the edge of their foot to help support it.
5. Add a little oil to your hands.
6. Slowly and gently separate their calf with the tips of your fingers. This involves gliding (page 24) to warm up the muscle, and then adding slower friction techniques (page 26) to isolate the muscle.
7. Perform the technique 3–5 times and increase the pressure a little each time.

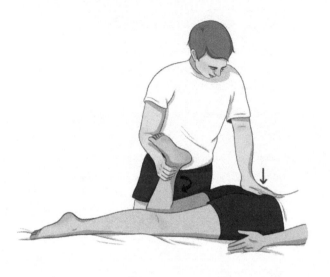

Gluteal Swivel

The gluteal region is associated with low back and leg pain, so it is a common focus area in sports massage. It's wonderful for loosening up the hip joint.

1. Your recipient is in the face down (prone) position.

2. Stand on one side of the table, and place your hand on the ball and socket joint (greater trochanter of the femur) closest to you.

3. Move the heel of your palm down and away from that area (the ball and socket are just used as a starting point).

4. Find a tender muscle area on the glutes and hold.

5. Lift the ankle of the same leg and slowly rotate and bend it from side to side (a few seconds each direction) while pressing down on the area on the glutes.

6. Continue the technique 20–30 seconds, and only to the recipient's desired pressure.

7. After you are done, find another tender area on the glutes and perform the technique again.

The Head Turner

By stretching a muscle and then massaging it, as you'll do in this technique, it's easier to apply more pressure and depth without straining your hands.

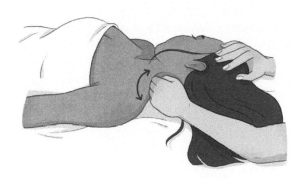

1. Your recipient is on their back (supine).
2. Slowly turn their head. Place one of your hands on their head for support.
3. Add a little oil on the knuckles of your other hand.
4. Slowly glide down (page 24) the back part of their neck.
5. Repeat 3–5 and increase the pressure a little each time.

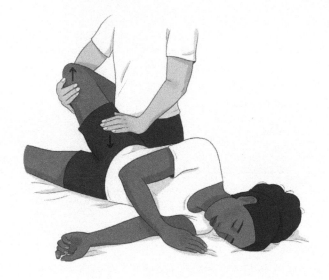

The TFL Abductor

The abductor muscles are muscles on the side of your hips (the TFL and vastus lateralis). The adductors are the inside leg muscles. This technique helps stretch out the adductors while massaging the abductors.

1. Have the recipient lie on their side.
2. Place your hand just below their hip bone on the TFL muscle (muscle on the side of their hip).
3. Keep holding the TFL muscle with one hand and place your other hand under their inside knee and slowly lift it up.
4. Lift their knee slowly for a few seconds, applying pressure to the TFL, and then bring the leg back to neutral.
5. Continue the technique 20–30 seconds, and only to the recipient's desired pressure.
6. After you are done, find another tender area on the abductor muscles and perform the method again.

Thai Massage

Thai massage is also called *nuad phaen boran Thai* or *Thai nuad*. Interestingly, Thai massage actually started in India. The founder of this style of massage is said to have been Shivago Komarpaj.

Just as *qi* is energy in China (and *ki* in Japan and *prana* in India), energy in Thailand is called *sen*. There are 10 sen lines (energy pathways flowing through your body) in Thai massage, though some people suggest there are thousands. Sen lines are similar to meridians in Traditional Chinese Medicine (page 13) and can become blocked in many ways—by injuries, trauma, stress, diseases, and other things. Thai massage techniques mainly focus on the sen lines to help heal ailments in the body.

The techniques in Thai massage are rhythmic pressing and stretching of the entire body. The practitioner uses their body in creative ways to increase the depth of the stretches and pressure. The body is compressed, pulled, stretched, and rocked during the treatment. It tends to be a deeper form of massage, so it's important to perform it slowly and within a person's pain tolerance. Thai massage uses no oils or lotions and is typically performed on the floor (you can do it on a massage table, but you have to make sure the table can support your weight and the weight of the receiver). The giver and receiver usually wear loose clothing.

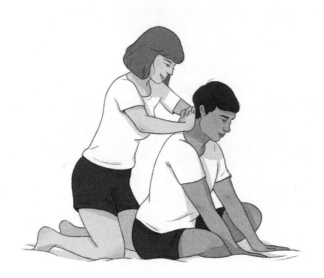

Compress My Neck

This technique is great for aiding relief to a stiff neck and headaches.

1. Have the recipient sit on the floor with their legs crossed and their hands on the floor in front of them supporting their body.

2. Kneel behind them so their neck is about at the height of your chest.

3. Interlock your fingers.

4. Squeeze the back portion of their neck between your palms.

5. Repeat 3–5 times in a rhythmic motion, slowly increasing pressure.

Hamstring/ Glute Stretch

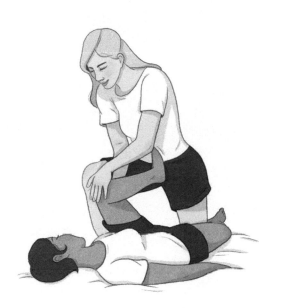

This move will stretch out the hamstrings and relieve some low back pain.

1. Have the recipient lie on their back (supine). Kneel next to them.

2. Flex one of their knees.

3. Place the foot of their bent leg on your hip bone.

4. Place one of your hands on their bent knee and the other on the calf.

5. Slowly press into their foot with your body, leaning your body toward their head.

6. You can use a rocking, rhythmic motion or a static stretch.

7. Repeat 3–5 times.

Prone Core Stretch

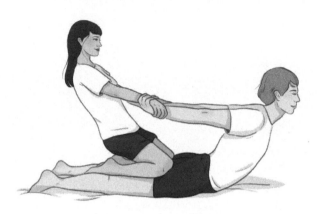

This is a big stretch for the shoulders and upper back and is great after spending the day hunched over a desk. It also helps stretch out the abdominal muscles.

1. Have the recipient lie face down (prone).
2. Place your feet between their knees and place your knees on their glutes. Make sure your body weight is even on both sides.
3. Interlock your wrists with their wrists.
4. Slowly lean back while pulling on their wrists to lift up their torso.
5. You can use a rocking, rhythmic motion or a static stretch.
6. Repeat 3–5 times.

Sitting Core Stretch

This is also another great stretch if you feel hunched over, just like the previous stretch. It's similar to the Prone Core Stretch, but you can place your feet up or down the back to get different stretches.

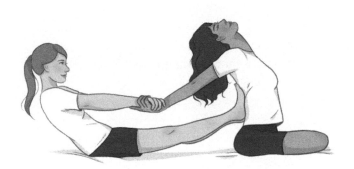

1. Have the recipient sit cross-legged.
2. Sit behind them and extend your legs, placing your feet in their mid-to-low back region.
3. Interlock your wrists with their wrists.
4. Slowly lean back while pushing your feet in their back and gently pulling their wrists.
5. You can use a rocking, rhythmic motion or a static stretch.
6. Repeat 3–5 times.

Tui Na

Tui na (pronounced "twee naw") is a form of Chinese massage therapy. The name comes from two of the actions used in the modality: *tui*, "to push," and *na*, "to lift and squeeze." It is related to Japanese massage or *anma*, the oldest-known form of traditional Asian massage. Tui na is a hands-on body treatment that uses Chinese Taoist principles to bring the eight principles of Traditional Chinese Medicine into balance.

This modality focuses a lot on acupressure points to help assist the healing process of people with acute and chronic musculoskeletal conditions (headaches, back pain and others), as well as many non-musculoskeletal conditions (PMS symptoms, insomnia and others). It incorporates shaking, tapotement, stretching, kneading, compression, and traction, along with other techniques. Tui na massage may be gentle or firm, and can be used on its own or in combination with acupuncture, fire cupping, moxibustion, Chinese herbalism, t'ai chi, or qigong.

8 PRINCIPLES OF TRADITIONAL CHINESE MEDICINE

1. **Yin:** Considered cold.
2. **Yang:** Considered heat.
3. **Interior:** Affects the internal organs and the bones.
4. **Exterior:** Affects skin, muscles, and energy meridians.
5. **Heat:** Symptoms can include a rapid pulse, fever, and dehydration.
6. **Cold:** Symptoms can include a tense pulse, body aches, and headaches.
7. **Deficiency:** Symptoms can include a slow pulse and constipation.
8. **Excess:** Symptoms can include a quick pulse and sharp stomach pains.

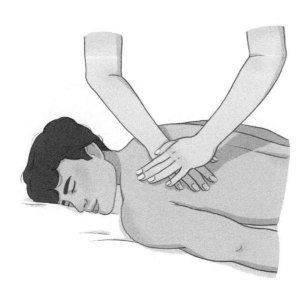

Vibration Technique

When performed for several seconds, this technique can be highly relaxing. It's similar to vibration in Swedish massage (page 28), but is usually performed with clothes on.

1. Place one of your hands over the other.

2. Vibrate quickly back and forth in that area for 5–10 seconds.

3. Go to another area of the body and repeat the technique sequence.

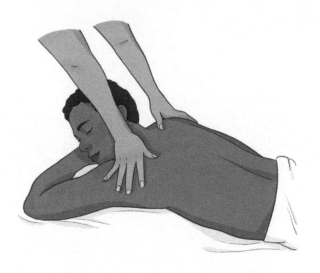

Kneading Technique

This technique is similar to petrissage (page 25), but it is usually performed with the person clothed. It helps reach all the layers of the muscles.

1. Place your thumbs on their back (1–2 inches away from their spine).
2. Use a circular motion with your thumbs in alternating directions.
3. Go to another area of the body and repeat the technique.

Quacking Technique

This technique penetrates all the layers of the muscles and is relaxing if performed fast and light. This technique should make a quacking sound.

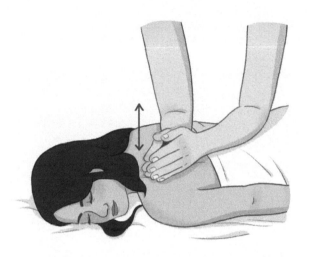

1. Place your hands together.
2. Strike the body with the side of your hands and make sure your hands are relaxed (avoid the spine and kidney region).

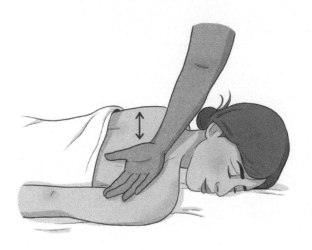

Padding Technique

This technique is similar to tapotement (page 27) but is usually performed with the person clothed.

1. Face your palm up.
2. Strike the body with a loose hand all around the back (avoid the spine and kidney region).

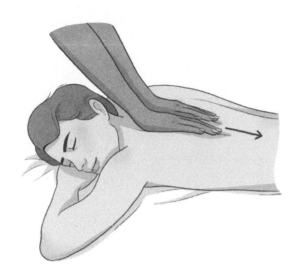

Pushing Technique

This technique is similar to effleurage (page 24), but you compress to get a good depth into the muscles before you glide your hands.

1. Place your hands on their back on each side of their spine.

2. Moderately push and glide your hands down their back (not on their spine).

3. Repeat 3–5 times.

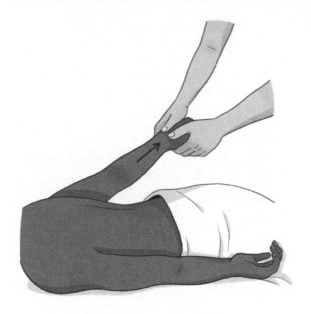

Pulling Technique

This is a form of stretching; check in with your recipient to make sure it's not too strong. The technique elongates the joint to stretch the joint more effectively.

1. Place your thumbs on the back of their wrist.

2. Have a firm grip and slowly pull.

3. You can hold the pull for 5–10 seconds and repeat if needed.

Ayurvedic

Ayurveda has been documented for millenia since around 5000 BCE. Ayurvedic massage focuses on marmas and chakras. In Ayurveda, marmas are vital points similar to acupressure points. There are more than a hundred vital marmas on the body. The seven great marmas in Ayurvedic massage are the same as the primary chakras (page 14). According to Ayurveda, each chakra aids organs and controls various aspects of our being. When chakras are blocked, dysfunction can occur in the body.

Ayurvedic massage techniques can be similar to Swedish massage, but tend to use more oil, faster motions, and not as much pressure as deep tissue massage.

THE DOSHAS: VATA, PITTA, AND KAPHA

In Ayurvedic tradition, the doshas are energies found throughout the human body and mind that when in balance contribute to total health and when out of balance, cause disruption or illness. In Ayurvedic medicine, health exists when there is a balance between the three doshas.

- **Vata** consists of the elements of space and air. It relates to the sinuses, nostrils, throat, bronchi, and lungs.
- **Pitta** consists of the elements fire and water. It relates to the liver, spleen, gallbladder, stomach, and pancreas.
- **Kapha** consists of the elements earth and water. It relates to the small and large intestines.

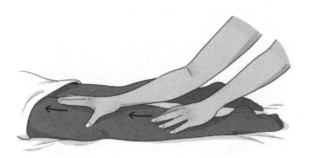

Fast Superficial Gliding

This technique is light and fast to help increase circulation and heat on the muscles. It can be used on the legs (anterior and posterior), arms (anterior and posterior), and back.

1. Add extra oil to your hands.

2. Glide (page 24) up and down the leg using a dynamic fast motion. This technique is usually performed twice as fast as regular gliding techniques, and at more of a superficial depth.

3. Repeat 3–5 times.

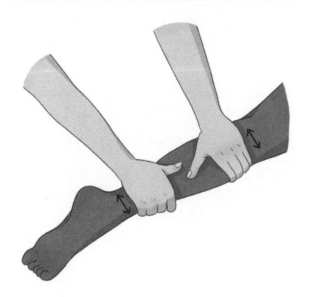

Invigorating Kneading

Usually with kneading techniques, I recommend less oil, but with this one, I like to add extra oil in order to perform it faster.

1. Add extra oil.
2. Move your hands back and forth in a vigorous motion while kneading and lifting up the muscles.
3. Repeat 3–5 times.

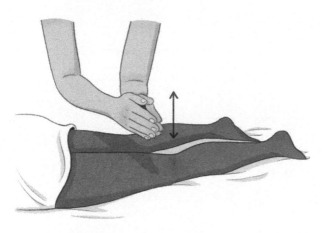

Hacking

This technique can be performed with a sheet on or with the skin exposed. It is a fast technique, which helps induce relaxation by adding rhythmic motions.

1. Place your hands together and strike the body with relaxed wrists/hands.

2. Start by lightly striking the body, and increase the depth and speed to the person's desire.

3. Do not perform over any bony areas, organs, or pulse regions.

4. Continue for 20–30 seconds.

Cranial Sacral

Craniosacral therapy (CST) is a form of treatment using a gentle touch or minimal pressure to palpate the joints of the skull, spine, and sacrum. This type of massage involves working with the craniosacral rhythm of the body to renew cerebrospinal fluid and is said to have many healing benefits.

Skilled practitioners work with still points, or pauses in the cranial sacral rhythm to find points of release. After the release, blood comes back into the area and circulation increases.

It is believed that craniosacral therapy helps the flow of cerebrospinal fluid, and thus helps induce a faster form of relaxation to the whole body. This modality is largely based on the work of two osteopathic physicians in the twentieth century. Dr. William Sutherland first practiced cranial osteopathy in the 1930s, and in the 1970s, Dr. John Upledger utilized Sutherland's earlier work to develop modern craniosacral therapy.

This modality uses around five grams of pressure (the weight of a nickel) and you can hold the pressure for 2–5 minutes. You may increase pressure slightly as you work.

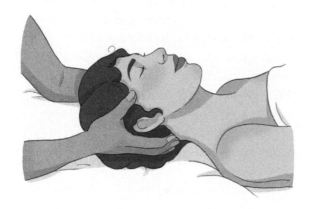

Sphenoid Bone Technique

This one of the core techniques of Cranial Sacral massage; it's a great way to start with this modality and helps induce relaxation. The sphenoid bone is located in the middle of the skull. Locate the temporal pulse, and it is just in front of it.

1. Have the recipient lie face up (supine).

2. Make an L shape with your hands.

3. Place all of your fingers behind their ears with your thumb in front of their ears.

4. Place your thumb on their sphenoid bone.

5. Apply the pressure of the weight of a nickel. Lightly hold for 2–5 minutes.

Occipital Base Technique

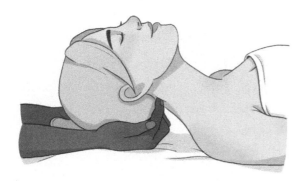

This technique is great for helping to relieve headaches.

1. Have the recipient lie face up (supine).

2. Hook your fingertips under the base of their head.

3. Allow the back of their head to rest on your palms.

4. Apply the pressure of the weight of a nickel. Lightly hold for 2–5 minutes.

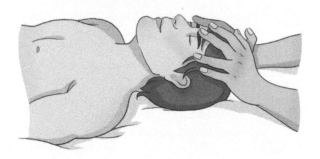

Frontal Bone Technique

The frontal bone is the bone on your forehead.

1. Have the recipient lie face up (supine).
2. Place your palms on the top of their head.
3. Place your fingers on their frontal bone.
4. Apply the pressure of the weight of a nickel. Lightly hold for 2–5 minutes.

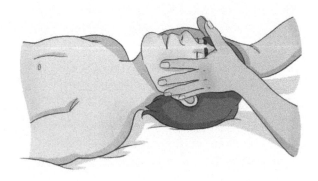

Mandible Bone Technique

1. Have the recipient lie face up (supine).

2. Place your palms on their temporal area (around the temples).

3. Place your fingers on their jaw.

4. Apply the pressure of the weight of a nickel. Lightly hold for 2–5 minutes.

Reflexology

Reflexology, originally known as zone therapy, is a modality that applies pressure to the feet and hands with thumb, finger, and hand techniques. It is based on a system of zones and reflex areas that purportedly reflect an image of the body on the feet and hands, with the premise that such work on the feet and hands affects a physical change to the rest of the body. You want to ask the receiver what problems they have in their body and then focus on the areas of the foot that correlate to those areas. For a generalized treatment, you would stimulate all parts of the foot.

While medical practices with marked similarities to zone therapy have existed for millennia, it was otolaryngologist William H. Fitzgerald who introduced zone therapy to the United States in 1913. Eunice D. Ingham, a physiotherapist, modified it the 1930s and 1940s. She was the first person to chart the body into "reflexes" on the feet. Her work continues to influence modern reflexology.

Reflexology can include the feet, hands, or both, though in this book I'll focus on the feet. Some reflexologists will not use any lubricant, and others will use cornstarch, oil, cream, or lotion—it's a matter of preference. Minimal lubricant allows you to apply direct pressure to the locations on the feet and hands and avoid slipping.

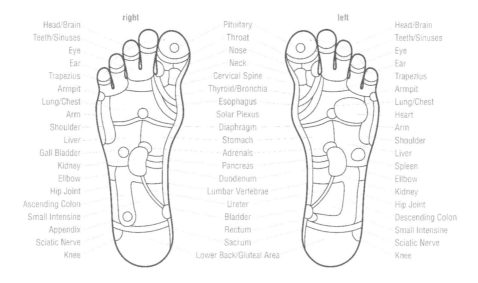

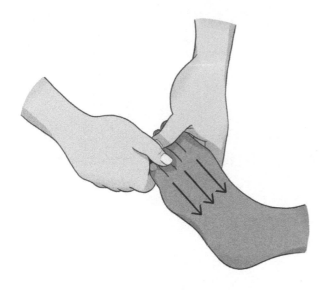

Between Tendon Slide

In reflexology, the top of the feet relate to the lung and chest. This technique can be tender on most people, so start out slow and with lighter pressure.

1. Slowly slide in between the tendons, one at a time.

2. You can increase pressure each time.

3. Repeat 3–5 times.

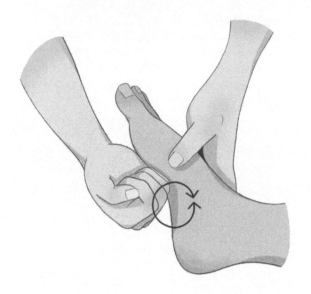

Knuckle Twist

With twisting techniques, you can increase pressure without adding more pressure to your technique.

1. Have one hand on top of their foot for support.
2. Make a fist with your other hand.
3. Place your knuckled grip on the bottom of their foot and move in a circular motion.
4. Increase the pressure a little each time, moving around the foot.

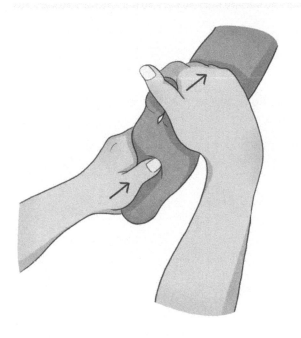

Compress & Extend

If someone wants more pressure, this is a great technique to use without adding any strain to your thumb. Instead, you're using their body to increase pressure.

1. Use one hand to hold their toes.

2. Place your thumb on the bottom of their foot and apply pressure.

3. Slowly extend their toes while keeping the pressure on the same spot on the bottom of the foot.

4. Repeat 3–5 times while flexing and extending their toes, all while keeping the same pressure. Find other tender areas in the foot and repeat 3–5 times in each area.

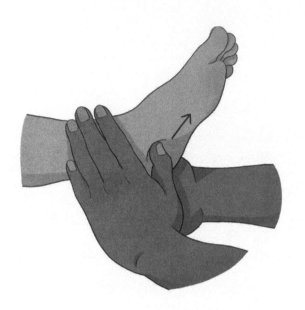

Inching

This technique helps you access all of the areas of the foot by moving an inch at a time. This technique can be used all over the foot and the toes.

1. Bend your thumb and then extend your thumb by gliding forward—roughly an inch each movement.

2. Repeat 3–5 times.

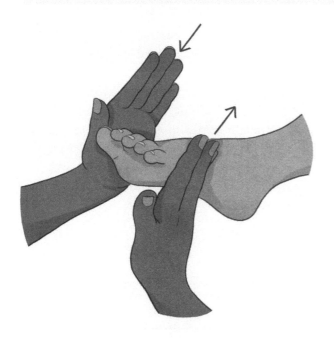

Shaky Foot

You can use this technique to gauge how relaxed your recipient is—the more movement they have, the more relaxed they are.

1. Place your hands on each side of their foot.

2. Move your hands back and forth slowly to start, rotating their foot in your hands.

3. Once you get a good rhythm, and the person begins to relax, increase the speed.

4. Continue for 20–30 seconds.

Reiki

Reiki is a modality that was developed in 1922 by Mikao Usui. It focuses on the seven main chakras (page 14), and it is based on *qi* (page 13), which is considered the universal life force in Traditional Chinese Medicine. The word reiki comes from the Japanese words "rei," which means "universal Life," and "ki," which means "energy." The practice of reiki can help balance the chakras.

A reiki session is usually performed entirely clothed. The techniques used are sometimes not even touching the body, or lightly placing your hands on specific chakras. Before you give any reiki treatment, it's important to ground yourself. Grounding is the process of ridding negative thoughts and replacing lost energy with energy from the earth. Some people imagine their feet as roots, continuing down into the earth to help focus during the session.

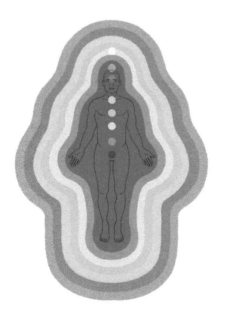

WHAT'S AN AURA?

An aura is a color emanation enclosing a body. The color of your aura is related to your physical, emotional, and spiritual health. Auras can be changed based on current mood, while your chakras are more stable. It takes real change in your life to create a change in your chakras. Reiki affects both auras and chakras.

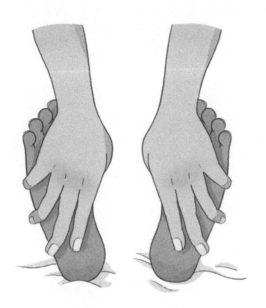

Grounding Technique

This is a great technique to help your recipient relax before you start.

1. Have the person lie face up (supine).

2. Either sit or stand at the side of the table.

3. Place both hands over the soles of their feet. You can hover over or place your hands on that area.

4. Hold for 30–60 seconds or until needed.

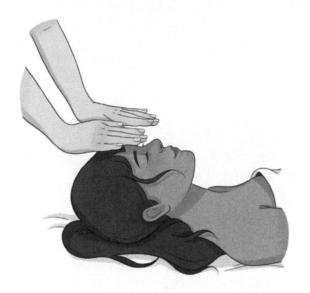

Third Eye Chakra

This helps with inner vision, intuition and wisdom.

1. Have the person lie face up (supine).

2. Either sit or stand at the head of the table.

3. Place your hands over their third eye chakra. You can hover over or place your hands gently on that area.

4. Hold for 30–60 seconds or until needed.

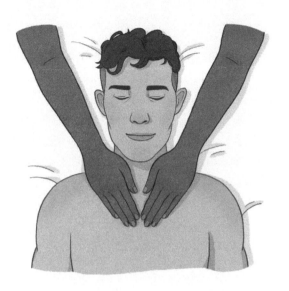

Throat Technique

This technique can help with communication and self-expression.

1. Have the person lie face up (supine).

2. Either sit or stand at the head of the table.

3. Place your hands over their throat chakra. You can hover over or place your hands on that area.

4. Hold for 30–60 seconds or until needed.

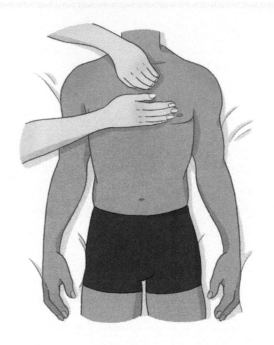

Heart Chakra

This technique can help with feelings of love and joy.

1. Have the person lie face up (supine).

2. Either sit or stand at the corner of the table.

3. Place both hands over their heart chakra. You can hover over or place your hands on that area.

4. Hold for 30–60 seconds or until needed.

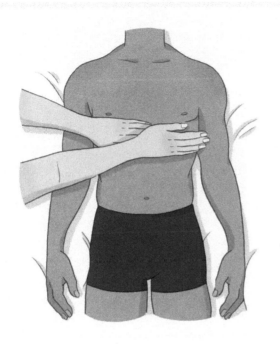

Solar Plexus Chakra

This practice helps with self-confidence and self-esteem.

1. Have the person lie face up (supine).

2. Either sit or stand at the side of the table.

3. Place both hands over their solar plexus chakra. You can hover over or place your hands on that area.

4. Hold for 30–60 seconds or until needed.

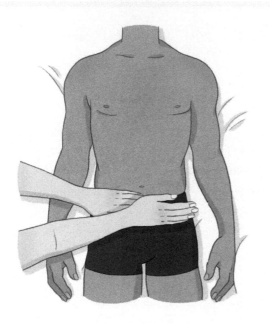

Sacral Chakra

This helps with pleasure and sexuality.

1. Have the person lie face up (supine).

2. Either sit or stand at the side of the table.

3. Place both hands over their sacral chakra. You can hover over or place your hands on that area.

4. Hold for 30–60 seconds or until needed.

Myofascial Release

Myo means "muscle," and "fascia" is a thin sheath of fibrous tissue enclosing a muscle or other organ (page 9). Myofascial release techniques are performed on the skin without oils, creams, or machines. This enables you to detect fascial restrictions accurately and apply the appropriate amount of sustained pressure to facilitate a release of the fascia. This helps improve flexibility of the fascia, muscles, and skin. Most techniques of myofascial massage focus on the superficial fascia, the lowermost layer of the skin in nearly all the regions of the body.

In this modality, you want to use relaxed hands; slowly stretching the fascia until it reaches a restriction. The length of time holding a stretch is usually 90 to 120 seconds. Myofascial release techniques are generally relaxing; typially it feels like a deep sustained stretch for the muscle.

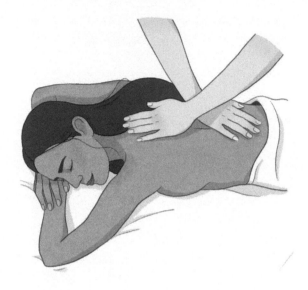

Cross Handed Stretch

This technique is easier to perform on the back and is widely seen in myofascial release pictures. It is great for larger areas of the body.

1. Have the person lie face up (supine).
2. Use no oil or lotion.
3. Cross your hands.
4. Let them sink into the muscles and fascia of the back.
5. Slowly push your hands out in opposite directions until you feel resistance.
6. Hold at that point for around two minutes, while still trying to stretch that area.

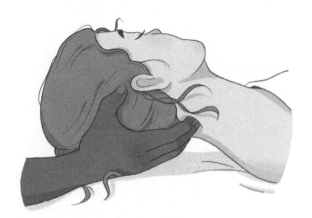

Suboccipital Stretch

This is one of the best techniques to help relieve headaches and relax the suboccipital muscles (the muscles right under the base of the skull), which are one of the main culprits of headaches.

1. Use no oil or lotion.
2. Hook your fingertips under the base of their skull.
3. Let them sink into the muscles and fascia.
4. Slowly separate your hands in opposite directions until you feel resistance.
5. Hold for around two minutes, while still trying to stretch that area.

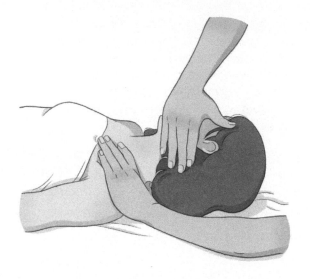

Neck Stretch

This technique helps release restrictions in the neck. It's great to use if someone wakes up with a stiff neck and has trouble turning their head.

1. Have the recipient lie face up (supine).

2. Use no oil or lotion.

3. Rotate their head to one side.

4. Place one hand at the bottom of their neck.

5. Place your other hand at their upper portion of their neck and jaw.

6. Slowly separate your hands in opposite directions until you feel resistance.

7. Hold for around two minutes, while still trying to stretch that area.

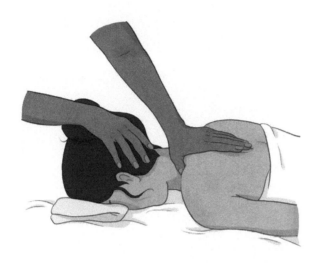

Posterior Neck Stretch

This is another great technique for relieving headaches, which often start in the back of your neck.

1. Have the person lie face down (prone). Use no oil or lotion.

2. Rotate their head to one side.

3. Hook your fingertips at the base of their skull.

4. Place your other hand on their upper shoulder.

5. Slowly separate your hands in opposite directions until you feel resistance.

6. Hold for around two minutes, while still trying to stretch that area.

CHAPTER 5

Massage for All

With over 200 different styles of massage out there, there's bound to be one that suits your needs. Now that you have a full repertoire, you can tailor your techniques to special life circumstances, such as a partner massage with your significant other or prenatal massage on an expectant mother.

The techniques in this chapter assume you're working with a generally healthy recipient. However, specific injuries, conditions, and diseases have certain precautions and contraindications (highly recommended not to massage). Always research this information before you give a massage to someone with a precaution or contraindication.

Partner Massage

A partner massage can be an intimate, bonding experience. It should never feel like a chore, and should be 50/50 in receiving and giving. Practice open communication and give honest, constructive feedback. A partners massage is an opportunity to get to know each other on a deeper level, both emotionally and physically. You can incorporate many techniques from the previous chapters into your couples massage. Below are some additional tips and tricks I've found to be helpful for couples new to massage.

Double Foot Massage

This is one of the best positions for couples because both couples receive and give at the same time, and can be face-to-face throughout the massage. It's also very comfortable.

1. Recline slightly on your backs facing each other on the couch. Have each person rest their feet on the other's chest.

2. You can use lotion or oils on each other's feet. Place a towel under your partner's feet if you are worried about getting oil on your clothes or the couch.

3. Massage for as long as desired, using a variety of massage techniques. I suggest placing your thumb on the bottom of their foot, and wrap your fingers over the top. Then, use circular friction (page 26) all over the bottom of their foot.

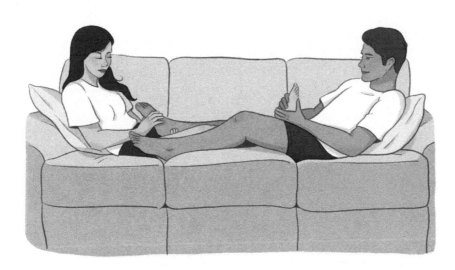

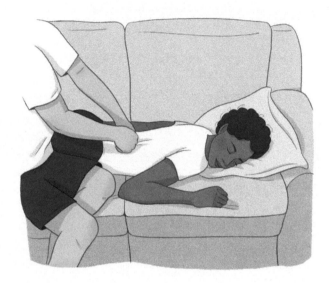

Massaging on a Couch #1

This tends to be a relaxing position for couples at home. When working on the couch, be sure to have the receiver turn their head to the other side every 5–10 minutes to prevent neck cramping.

1. Have the receiver lie face down on the couch, and the giver kneel beside their hips. If the receiver has back problems, place a pillow under their ankles to relax the hamstring muscles.

2. Mix and match styles and techniques, and massage as long as you desire before switching places. If you're comfortable, have the receiver remove their shirt and the giver use oil or lotion to perform more gliding techniques (page 24).

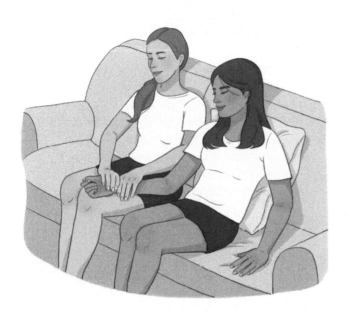

Massaging on a Couch #2

This is a relaxed, casual position where the couple is sitting side-by-side. You can easily carry on a conversation if that fits the mood, or just enjoy being together in the quiet while performing this massage.

1. Sit side-by-side on the couch. If you are worried about getting lotion or oil on your couch, place a towel under the receiver's hand.

2. Massage the hand and arm that is close to you. Snake Bite (page 49) works great in this position, as well as kneading (page 25).

3. When you're done with that side, move to the other side to massage the other hand and arm. Mix styles and techniques as desired before switching roles.

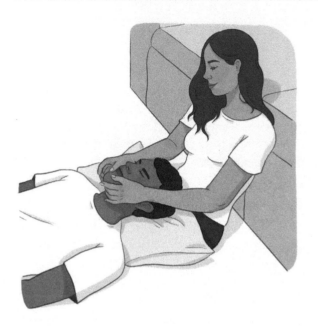

Massaging on a Couch #3

This position is a great hack if you don't have a massage table. It's also more intimate, so perfect for couples. Most people do not want any oil on their face when receiving a massage, but check if lotion is okay. If the recipient has a beard, use more finger pressure and either circular motions or compression (page 30) to prevent pulling the hairs.

1. Have the giver sit against a wall or the couch with their legs relaxed out in front of them, and have them place a pillow in their lap. This protects the receiver's neck.

2. Have the receiver lie down on their back with their head propped up on the pillow.

3. Start by gliding (page 24) around the face with your fingertips or with your thumbs on their forehead.

4. Continue gently massaging the face before swapping places.

Massaging in a Chair

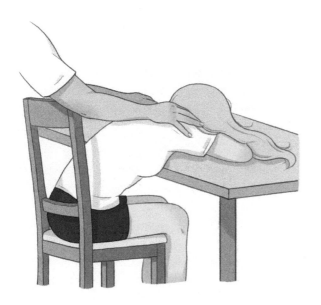

This is an easy hack for giving a proper neck or shoulder massage if you don't have a massage table. Make sure to turn the chair sideways (or use an open-backed chair) so the giver can easily access the back.

1. Place a pillow on a table or desk. Have the receiver lie their head and shoulders on the pillow with their arms loosely bent and relaxed on the table.

2. Have the giver stand to massage the back, neck, and shoulders, mixing styles and techniques to their preference. If the receiver feels comfortable, they can remove their shirt and you can use oil or lotion to perform more gliding techniques.

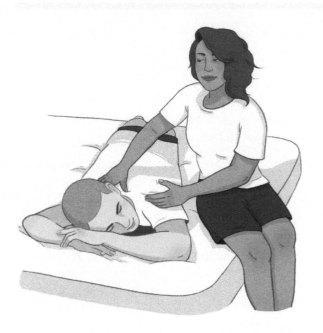

Massaging on a Bed

Massaging on the bed is great to do before winding down your day and tucking in. If you use oil or lotion on bare skin, place a towel under the receiver to protect your bedding. You can massage all posterior areas of the body in this position.

1. Have the receiver lie face down on the bed. Make sure they move to one side of the bed, so the giver doesn't have to lean over too much. Have the giver sit beside one shoulder.

2. Massage the shoulders and upper and lower back using a blend of techniques and styles. If you're comfortable, have the receiver remove their shirt and the giver can use oil or lotion to perform more gliding techniques (page 24).

3. To switch sides, have the giver move to the other side of the bed and resume the position.

Prenatal Massage

When someone is pregnant, their body goes through many changes. They can experience different kinds of pain and discomfort than what they may have in the past, or even in past pregnancies. Every pregnancy is different. I know this firsthand, as I have two kids, and massaged my wife throughout both of her pregnancies. In each pregnancy, there were different and distinct areas that she needed massaged.

Massage helps the parent-to-be relax and eases their aches and pains. Be sure to ask for lots of feedback to make sure the techniques feel good. It's possible their needs will change week by week (or even day to day!) so always check in. Prenatal massage is a wonderful source of comfort during pregnancy, and can help couples bond, too.

In the second and third trimester, the best position for massaging the back is having the recipient lie on their side. If their legs, arms, and face need massage, lying on the back with an elevated head works best. Always start with lighter pressure and slowly increase the pressure to their desire. If there have been any complications, it's essential to consult their physician before trying massage.

BASIC PRECAUTIONS FOR PRENATAL MASSAGE

Below is a list of basics for areas to avoid or approach with caution when someone is pregnant. If there's ever a concern, consult a medical professional.

- **Ankles and wrists:** In reflexology, these areas are connected to the ovaries and uterus, so it is best to avoid sustained deep pressure in these areas.
- **Abdominal Area:** It's okay to use very light, gentle pressure on the abdomen area.
- **Deep pressure on the legs:** Because pregnancy increases risk of blood clots or poorer circulation, techniques on the legs should be gentler and more relaxing.
- **Never massage the pelvic region:** This is true not only for prenatal massage, but for every type of massage and technique.

Side-Lying Back Massage

This is a very comfortable position, especially for the second and third trimesters. The pillows add additional support. The recipient flips to the other side halfway through the massage to massage some of the harder to reach places.

1. Have the recipient lie on one side and hug a pillow. Place one pillow under their head, and one between their knees to keep their hips aligned.

2. Add oil to your hands.

3. Slowly glide (page 24) up and down their back, avoiding the spine. Increase the pressure to their desire. Kneading techniques (page 25) also work well for this position.

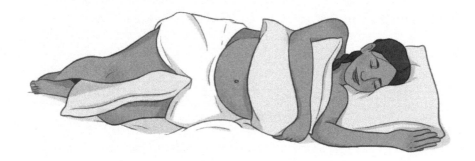

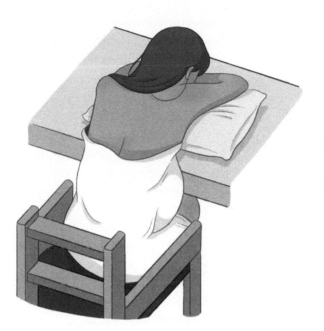

Sitting Back Massage

1. Have the recipient sit in a chair, preferably one with a low or open back. You can also turn the chair to the side. Place a pillow on top of the table and have them lightly hug it while resting their chin on the pillow.

2. If their back is bare, start by adding oil to your hands.

3. Knead their shoulders in a circular motion. Continue this technique for 20–30 seconds, and increase the pressure to her desire. You can also use compression techniques (page 30) along the spine.

Baby Massage

Baby massage is an excellent way for parents to bond with their baby. It can be beneficial for both the parents and the baby. One groundbreaking study from Dr. Tiffany Field shows that massaging babies born prematurely can increase their weight gain, which can help them recover faster and limit their hospital stay. Parents benefit from the bonding experience.

Baby massage started to gain popularity in the early 1970s. Now there are instructors all over the world who teach baby massage techniques to new parents. Parents typically don't bring their baby in for a professional massage, because you don't know if they will accept a massage from someone else. It's a lot easier for a parent to perform the massage on the baby's own terms. Plus, it helps with bonding and connection.

BABY MASSAGE PRECAUTIONS

It's best to massage your baby on the floor on a blanket, or on your lap while you sit on the floor. This is safest for your baby. Avoid high surfaces like tables, changing tables, or beds. A bed can be okay as long as they can't roll over, are placed safely in the center of the bed, and you stay with them the whole time.

Gentle pressure is recommended. Since a baby can't express their exact needs, you may want to spend 20–30 minutes massaging their body all over and seeing how it goes.

Never, ever force your baby to receive a massage. If they are not in the mood for one, they will let you know. You can ease them into accepting a massage by singing to them, talking in a calm voice, or playing with them to test the waters.

Use jojoba oil or grape-seed oil. These work well for babies because they don't have scents. Never add essential oils used for aromatherapy to the massage oil, because babies tend to put their hands in their mouth. Typically 10–20 minutes is ideal for an infant massage, but it all depends on what the infant can handle.

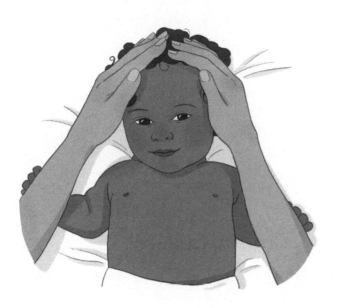

Baby Face Massage

This technique is a great, gentle way to start out the massage. Your baby will feel safe because they can see your face and everything that you're doing.

1. Place your baby face up on a blanket on the floor.

2. Rub your hands back and forth to warm them up.

3. Place your hands on their face and scalp without any oil.

4. Slowly glide (page 24) around their face avoiding their eyes.

5. Continue the technique 20–30 seconds.

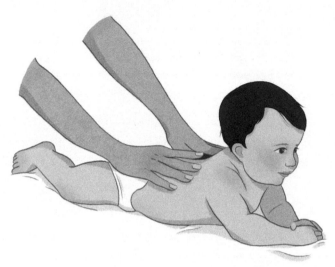

Baby Back Massage

1. Place your baby face down on a blanket on the floor.

2. Add olive oil or grape-seed oil to your hands.

3. Slowly glide (page 24) up and down their back, avoiding their spine.

4. Continue the techniques for 20–30 seconds. Maintain very gentle pressure without increasing too much.

Stomach Massage

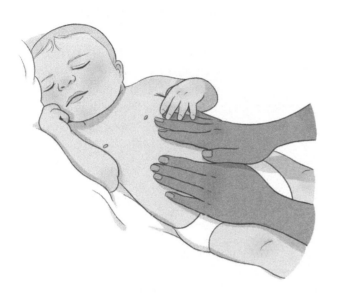

This technique is great for colicky babies, because massage can help soothe their stomach and intestinal discomfort.

1. Place your baby face up on a blanket on the floor.

2. Add jojoba oil or grape-seed oil to your hands.

3. Slowly glide (page 24) your fingertips around their belly in a clockwise circular motion.

4. Continue the technique for 20–30 seconds.

Senior Massage

My absolute favorite population to massage is seniors. I genuinely love hearing their stories, even if they've told me the same story many times. I first started working in a nursing home when I was seventeen years old. It had its ups and downs, but helping out was gratifying. While I was going to massage school, I asked some of the residents if I could practice on them, and they all loved it.

Now working in a hospital, I still get the opportunity to massage seniors—I see a lot of them in the medical surgical unit. I massage a lot of patients who have had knee or hip replacements, gastrointestinal issues, respiratory problems, and other issues. With patients being in their recovery room for 2–3 days on average, massage is an excellent way to relieve some of their pain and increase their circulation.

With Baby Boomers being the most significant aging population in the United States, as a professional, it makes sense to get skilled in massaging seniors now. An added bonus is that they can teach you so much by just massaging them. At home, this can be a great way to connect with and learn from your older relatives.

SENIOR MASSAGE PRECAUTIONS

There are some precautions to consider when massaging seniors. If someone has a specific condition, such as calf pain with heat, open sores, osteoporosis, or other specific needs, be sure to do more research and speak to a doctor before massaging them.

One important thing to remember is that it can be difficult for an older adult to lie on their stomach. The best positions for seniors are face up (supine), side lying, or sitting in a chair. If they seem frail, then 30–45 minutes is more than enough for a massage. If they are stronger and want a longer massage, then 60–90 minutes is perfectly fine. I use massage gel or oil because the skin of most seniors is dry and tends to need as much moisture as possible. Lotion is okay, but it absorbs too fast.

When I worked in nursing homes, sometimes the residents would be on comfort care, which sadly means the end of their life is near. When caring for these individuals, do whatever you can to make them comfortable.

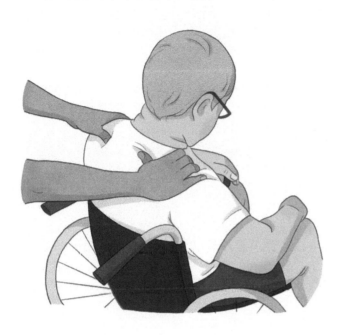

Chair Massage for Shoulders

For some seniors, it is not advisable for them to lie face down on a massage table. Sitting in a chair allows you to access their back, neck, shoulders, scalp, arms, and hands.

1. Have them sit in their wheelchair or a regular chair if they're able. You can have them seated at a table and place a pillow between their chest and table, allowing them to lean on the pillow so they feel more stable.

2. Ask them take a few deep breaths before you begin.

3. Place your hands on their shoulders and slowly knead (page 25) their muscles in a circular motion. Continue with this technique for 20–30 seconds, and increase the pressure to their desire.

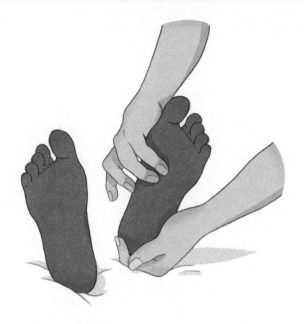

Face up Massage for Feet

Massaging the feet and hands of a senior can be very beneficial, especially if they have arthritis.

1. Ask them if you can remove their socks, or if they prefer to do it themselves. Have them lie face up on a bed. Elevate their head with a pillow if it's hard for them to lie flat on their back or to breathe in this position.

2. Add some lotion or oil to your hands. Hold their foot in your hands for 5–10 seconds to help them get used to your touch and dissipate the ticklish sensation.

3. Slowly knead (page 25) their feet in a circular motion, increasing the pressure to their desire.

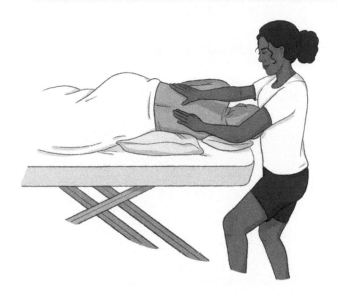

Side Lying Back Massage

For some seniors, lying on their stomach for a back massage is not doable. Side lying is a great alternative, as it provides more comfort for them while still giving you access to the whole back.

1. Ask them which side they feel more comfortable lying on.

2. Add oil or lotion to your hands.

3. Slowly glide up and down their back, but avoid their spine.

4. Use circular friction (page 26) motions with your thumbs along the side of their spine and around their shoulders.

5. Perform each technique for 30–60 seconds all over their back and increase the pressure to their desire.

CHAPTER 6

Healing with Massage

Now that you have a thorough understanding of massage techniques, styles, and positions, you can focus on healing specific ailments or pains with massage. Remember, two of the main reasons people seek massage are they are stressed or they have pain. When they are stressed, a soothing, light-to-medium pressure massage throughout the body helps relax them. When people are in pain, they typically want more focus on the problem area.

When it comes to healing, you can incorporate different methods that are not related to massage. You don't need an expensive spa to get the full healing experience. All the methods are easy and inexpensive to recreate at home. For instance, try using warm oil (you can buy bottle warmers at massage supply stores) and warm towels (you can purchase a towel warmer, or use a large slow cooker) to help relax muscles a lot faster. This feels wonderful for the recipient, and means you'll spend less time warming the muscles up before adding more pressure. Aromatherapy, which generally costs extra at a spa, is easy to add to your home practice for a fraction of the price. Incorporating stretching into a message is also a wonderful manual healing technique.

Essential Oils

Essential oils are concentrated aromatic compounds extracted from plants. These natural scents are believed to have both physical and psychological healing benefits. Essential oils are used in a variety of products from massage oil, incense, hair products, skincare products and more.

An aromatherapist is someone who specializes in the practice of aromatherapy. They mix essential oils that can be used through topical application or inhalation. When starting out, you may want to consult an aromatherapist and get recommendations for the best oils to use for certain ailments. I've also provided a preliminary list of my favorite healing oils below.

There are two ways to use essential oils in massage: inhalation and topical application. For inhalation, you can use a diffuser, steam inhalation, baths, or put some drops on a cotton ball and have the recipient breathe in the scent. If you're applying topically, remember that people can have reactions to essential oils applied directly to the skin. Therefore, it's important to add essential oils to a *carrier oil*, which dilutes the essential oil and "carries" it to the skin. Jojoba oil and grape-seed oil are common carrier oils. Always ask the recipient if they want essential oils or if they are allergic to them.

Essential oils are sold at a range of prices, and price point is generally a good indicator of quality. Rose essential oil is one of the most expensive, because it takes a lot of roses to get the essential oil from the petals. Citrus essential oils are cheaper, because it doesn't take as much citrus to make an ounce. I recommend trying a few different brands and seeing which you like best.

Light can affect the properties of the oils, so always buy essential oils sold in dark-colored bottles.

CARRIER OILS

Using carrier oils is ideal when making your aromatherapy massage oil. In addition to making the oils safer for the skin, it makes your essential oils last longer.

Typically you want to add 10–20 drops of essential oil to an 8-ounce bottle of carrier oil. Less is always better to start; you can always add more if desired.

Carrier oils can be purchased at natural grocery stores and are generally reasonably priced. The popular carrier oils are:

- **Jojoba oil:** Provides a nice glide with your massage techniques.

- **Grape-seed oil:** Absorbs more quickly so you can perform deeper techniques without slipping on the muscles.

- **Fractionated coconut oil:** The liquid form of the coconut and won't solidify like regular coconut oil. This carrier oil is the best one to use when adding essential oils, because the carrier oil absorbs quickly, meaning the body can quickly benefit from the healing properties of the essential oils.

Other carrier oils include sweet almond, apricot kernel, avocado, calendula, evening primrose, and sesame.

ESSENTIAL OIL PRECAUTIONS

Here are a few precautions to keep in mind as you begin working with essential oils.

- Never ingest essential oils. Some are extremely poisonous.

- If you are working with someone who is pregnant, it is important for them to consult a physician before using essential oils on their skin.

- If someone has skin diseases, they should talk to their physician to see if they can safely use essential oils on their skin.

- Some oils can have a negative reaction when combined with certain prescription medications. If someone is on meds, have them talk to their doctor about possible reactions before using essential oils.

- Exposure to UV light can cause a reaction if you have certain essential oils on your skin. Wash off these essential oils before going into direct sunlight.

- Always keep essential oils out of the reach of children. They are powerful substances and should be treated as such.

TOP ESSENTIAL OILS FOR MASSAGE

Below are some of the most popular essential oils
and their believed healing benefits:

Basil: A peppery essential oil, it can help with sore muscles, breathing, and fatigue.

Bergamot: A citrus and floral-tinged oil used to flavor Earl Grey tea, it can help with anxiety, body weight, and heart health.

Black pepper: A warm and spicy essential oil that can help detoxify and alleviate anxiety.

Cinnamon: This oil helps with infections, inflammation, and skin problems.

Eucalyptus: With a sharp, fresh scent, it can help with coughs, breathing, and congestion.

Frankincense: This oil has a lovely woodsy and spicy smell. It can help with inflammation, memory, and building immunity.

Geranium: A sweet-smelling essential oil. It can help with acne, inflammation, and anxiety.

Ginger: A spicy and sharp-scented essential oil with a hint of lemon and pepper, it can help with inflammation, joints, digestion, and nausea.

Grapefruit: Sharp, tart, and refreshing, grapefruit essential oil can help with concentration and metabolism.

Lavandin: A light and floral essential oil. It can help with scars, stretch marks, and circulation, and is also used for cleaning.

Lavender: A very popular essential oil, lavender can help with anxiety and insomnia.

Lemon: This can kill bacteria and help with oily hair. Lemon is the most common essential oil used in cleaning products.

Lemon balm: A lemony and minty essential oil, it can help with menopause, insomnia, and memory.

Lemongrass: This oil has a sweet, lemony scent and can help with muscle pain and digestion, and is even used as a bug repellant.

Lime: This citrus has a sharp and sweet scent. It can help with concentration, digestion, and repelling bugs.

Marjoram: Warm and spicy, this oil can help circulation, muscle pain, and breathing.

Myrrh: This is a musky essential oil. It can help with infections and inflammation.

Orange: Sweet, tangy, and refreshing, orange oil can help with colds, flu, and healing wounds.

Patchouli: With its musky and spicy smell, this one is a classic. It can help with constipation, wounds, inflammation, and anxiety.

Peppermint: With a fresh menthol scent, this oil can help with nausea, upset stomachs, gas, anxiety, and pain.

Roman chamomile: This is a sweet, apple-scented essential oil. It can help with inflammation, burns, bruises, and insomnia.

Rose: Smelling of fresh roses, this essential oil can help with anxiety.

Rosemary: With an earthy, herbal scent, rosemary oil can help thicken hair and improve memory.

Sage: Sharp and herbal, sage can help with digestion, inflammation, and symptoms of PMS.

Sandalwood: With a woodsy and exotic scent, sandalwood oil can help increase libido.

Spearmint: This oil has a minty and sweet smell. It can help with breathing and stress.

Tea tree: Spicy and pungent, this oil can help with coughs and wounds.

Ylang-ylang: Sweet and exotic smelling, this oil can help with blood pressure and relaxation, and can increase libido.

Low Back Pain

Low back pain is one of the most common physical problems. It's estimated that 80 percent of Americans will have an episode of low back pain within their lifetime. Most people think that low back pain is only located in the low back, but that's not the case for everyone. Nerve injuries, poor posture, weak abdominal muscles, and buttocks pain can all contribute to low back pain.

I like to place warm or hot towels on the low back before massaging the area, to help warm up the muscles.

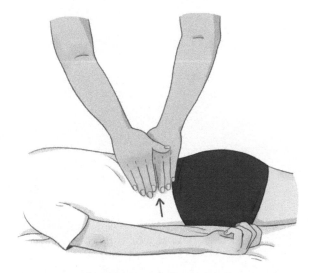

Low Back Lift

This technique helps control how much pressure is used on a tender low back. If it's too much pressure the hip will lower slowly, and if it's not enough pressure, it will lower too fast.

1. Have the recipient lie face down (prone). Stand by one of their hips, and ask them to lift the opposite hip as high as they can.

2. Place your hands on their opposite hip and low back.

3. Have them slowly push their hip down onto the table while you add pressure to their low back region and glide (page 24) your hands to the center of their back. Stop just before you reach their spine.

4. Repeat 3–5 times and increase the pressure a little more each time.

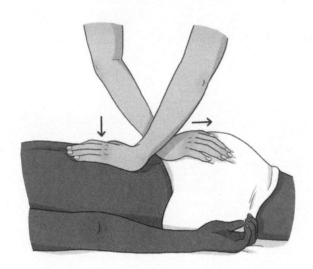

Elongate the Low Back

This is a gentle massage technique that works well for relieving lower back pain.

1. Have the recipient lie face down (prone). Stand beside one of their hips.

2. Place your supporting hand just above the hip closest to you, but don't add too much pressure on their bone (this can cause bruising).

3. Add a little oil to your other hand.

4. Start at their lower back and slowly glide (page 24) from their lower back to their midback.

5. Repeat 3–5 times, increasing the pressure a little more each time.

Ratcheting the Glutes

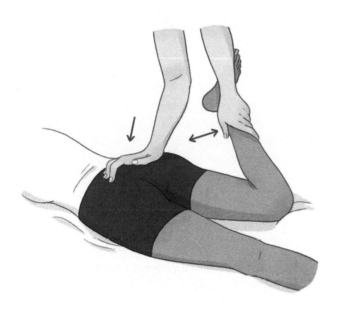

Just below the hip bone is the gluteus medius, a muscle can cause low back pain. Therefore, it's important to not just massage the area of pain, but all around that area.

1. Have the recipient lie face down (prone). Stand on one side by their hip.

2. Place the heel of your hand on their buttock (the upper portion, just below their hip).

3. Find a tender muscle area on their buttocks and then lift up the foot of that same leg.

4. Keep the pressure on their buttocks and slowly move their foot back and forth for a few seconds each direction. Maintain the same amount of pressure with the heel of your hand.

5. Check in with them and only bring the discomfort to a 6 out of 10.

6. Continue this technique for 20–30 seconds, and then move to another area on the buttocks.

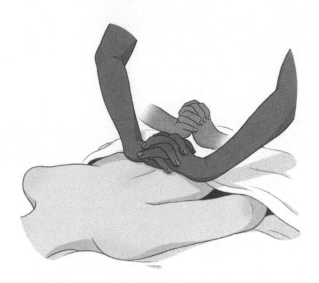

Lower Back Press

Some people might be cautious about lower back massages, because they are concerned that you might hit their kidneys (the truth is that you have to go really deep to do that). With this technique, you can assure them that won't happen. This move directly targets the lower back muscle on the sides of the spine.

1. Have the recipient lie face down (prone).
2. It is best not to use any extra oil with this technique.
3. Interlock your fingers.
4. Place the heels of your palms on each side of their lower back and just push into the muscles on the side of their spine. Be careful not to slip.
5. Squeeze and hold 10-20 seconds.

Forearm Pain

There are many possible causes of forearm pain. Some react well to deeper work, while other conditions may only tolerate lighter pressure. With this technique you can apply more or less pressure as needed. One area in particular where you want to avoid applying deeper pressure is the median nerve, which is located directly in the center of the inner forearm on the flexor area.

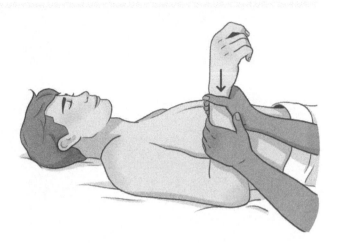

Gravity

With this technique, you access the full forearm and apply pressure as needed.

1. Have the recipient lie face up (supine).
2. Place their triceps on the table while lifting up their hand.
3. Add oil to your hand and have them hold their hand up the whole time.
4. Cup their forearm with your hands and slowly slide down their forearm all the way to their elbow. Use compression (page 30) and deep friction (page 26).
5. Repeat 3–5 times, and increase the pressure each time to their desire.

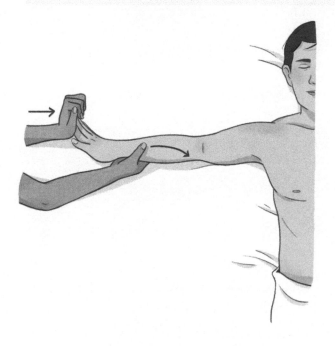

Wrist Bar

This technique helps you isolate every inch of the forearm to find and treat discomfort.

1. Extend their wrist and place your other hand and thumb on their lower arm (just above their wrist).

2. Slowly flex their wrist while sliding your thumb up their forearm, all the way to just before their elbow.

3. Repeat 3–5 times, asking for feedback on the pressure level, and increase the pressure each time to their desire.

PMS

PMS is associated with many physical symptoms like fatigue, cramping, bloating, and lower back pain. This technique can be really helpful for lower back pain.

While it may seem counterintuitive, do not massage the stomach (abdominal) region. Instead, focus more on the glutes and lower back to relieve pressure in the lower back. I like to use essential oils: eucalyptus, lavender, ylang-ylang, Roman chamomile, and geranium are all good options.

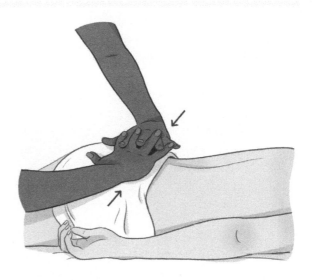

Compress PMS

Massaging the glute region usually has the most benefits for PMS symptoms. Compressing the sides of the sacrum can help relieve cramping sensations.

To find the sacrum, locate the lower spine then follow it past the hips. It's directly in the center of the buttocks right above the tailbone (coccyx).

1. Have the recipient lie face down (prone).
2. Stand beside them and interlock your fingers.
3. Place the heel of your palms on the sides of their sacrum.
4. Squeeze into the sacrum and hold for 10–20 seconds.
5. Repeat 3–5 times, and increase the pressure to their desire.

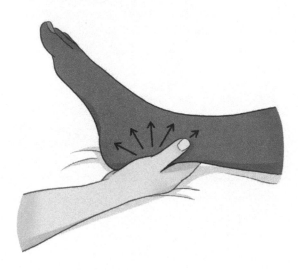

Sun

In reflexology (page 110), the area around the ankles relates to the lower abdominal area. Therefore, it's believed that massaging the ankle can help relieve PMS symptoms.

1. Have them seated and place their foot out in front of them on a table.

2. Add a little oil or lotion to your hands.

3. Slowly glide (page 24) your thumb in different gliding directions radiating out from the ankle (like beams from the sun).

4. Repeat 3–5 times in each direction, and increase the pressure to their desire. This technique can be performed on each side of the ankle, and on both legs.

Knee Pain

Knee pain is more common in serious athletes, weekend warriors, and older adults. If you are massaging the area that has pain, you could be in the wrong place because trigger points (as stated in chapter one, page 6) typically refer pain to other areas.

One area to focus on is just above the knee on their quad muscles, because trigger points on the quadriceps can refer pain to the knee. Be careful not to massage directly on the kneecap; it's best not to push the kneecap around. When a person's leg is lying on a table with their leg straight, their kneecap will move around. When the knee is bent, you're less likely to move the kneecap.

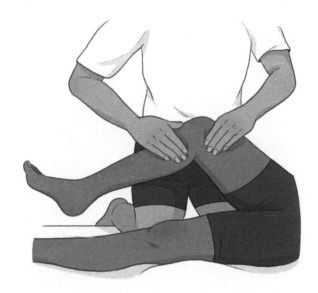

Knee Lift

This technique helps you locate trigger points above and below the knee, which can refer pain to their kneecap. As you massage around the knee, ask if they have any referred pain.

1. Have the recipient lie face up (supine). Put one of your knees on the table near their knee. Lift up their knee and place their calf on your quads.
2. Add a little oil or lotion to your hands.
3. Squeeze above and below their knee with your fingers and thumbs.
4. Slowly slide off those areas.
5. Repeat 3–5 times, and increase the pressure to their desire.

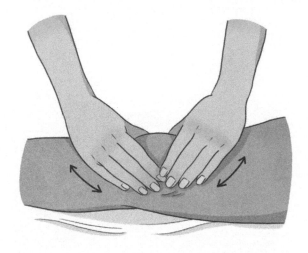

Kneecap Friction

Make sure their knee and leg are flat on the table before you begin. Friction around the kneecap can help increase range of motion and break up scar tissue.

1. Have the recipient lie face up (supine).

2. Add a little oil or lotion to your hands.

3. Friction (page 26) around their kneecap (patella) and use slow gliding techniques (page 24) using your fingertips or thumbs.

4. Continue this technique for 20–30 seconds on each side of the kneecap and increase the pressure to their desire.

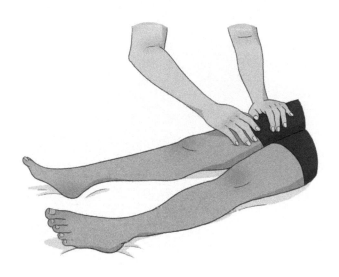

Knead Quad

The quadriceps muscles typically refer pain to the knee. Relieving these muscles can also help treat knee pain.

1. Have the recipient lie face up (supine).
2. Place a little oil or lotion on your hands.
3. Knead (page 25) the quad muscles, like you are kneading bread.
4. Continue a circular kneading motion all over the quadriceps muscles.
5. Continue this for 20–30 seconds in one specific area, then perform it again on other areas of the quads.

Headaches and Neck Pain

Headaches are a common reason people seek out massage. Massage can be beneficial for headaches by slowly massaging the shoulders and back of the neck. The slower you go, the less likely the recipient will feel much discomfort during the process.

Another complaint I hear a lot is a stiff neck. People will wake up with pain and tightness in the neck and complain that it is hard to turn their neck. Hunching over a computer or mobile device can also cause neck and shoulder pain. When massaging someone with a stiff neck, make sure you never force a stretch and always communicate about the discomfort.

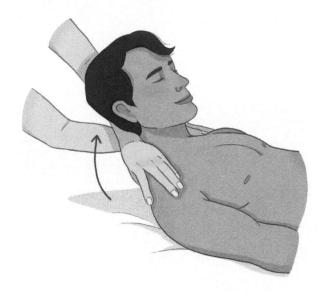

Neck Flex

This technique helps relax the neck muscles, which almost anyone can benefit from, considering how much time we spend looking down at our phones these days!

1. Have the recipient lie face up (supine).
2. Cross your forearms and place your hands on the opposite shoulders.
3. Slowly lift their neck with your forearms while compressing their shoulders with your hands.
4. Once they feel the stretch, hold it for 20–30 seconds.

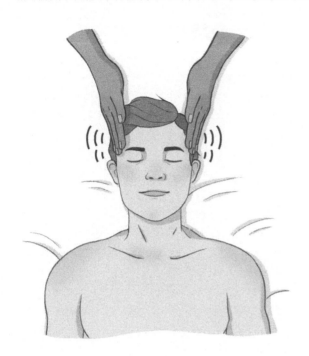

Temple Turn

Circular rhythmic motions can be relaxing when performed for 10–20 seconds.

1. Have the recipient sitting up or lying face up.

2. Do not add any oil or lotion to your hands.

3. Place your fingertips on their temple region.

4. Slowly rotate your fingertips without adding a lot of pressure.

5. Continue the technique for 10–20 seconds.

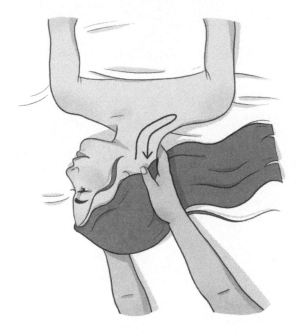

Can't Hear

It's common for headaches to start in the neck. This technique accesses the whole neck and is good for relieving headaches, a stiff neck, or both.

1. Have the recipient lie face up (supine).

2. Slowly bring their neck to their right side, and then rotate their head until their right eye is on the table (or as far as they can comfortably turn their head).

3. Add oil to your right hand and place your left hand under their neck for support.

4. Glide (page 24) down the left side of their neck with your hand using light pressure, going around their shoulder.

5. Then, increase the pressure a little more and you glide up the back part of their shoulder and neck.

6. Stop at the base of their skull and hold 5–10 seconds (not on their spine).

7. Repeat this technique 3–5 times, and increase the pressure to their desire. Then repeat on the other side.

Foot Pain

If you are on your feet all day long at your job, then you probably understand foot pain and the need for a great foot massage. Using a compression (holding) technique (page 30) can help diffuse some of the ticklishness sensation, and using essential oils can be very therapeutic. If the recipient is very shy about having their feet touched, you can always tell them that you're happy to massage their feet with their socks on.

The two areas on the feet to which people tend to want more attention paid are the heels and arches. With heels, which are typically fairly tough, you need to add a little more pressure. You can also use your knuckles to increase the depth of pressure.

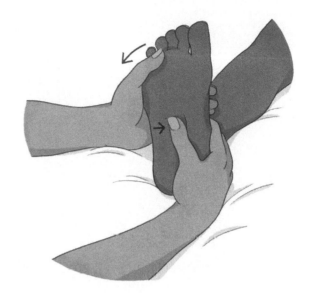

Rotate Out – Slide In

Rotating the foot before gliding makes it easier for to increase pressure while still being effective at pinpointing their pain.

1. Add oil or lotion to your right hand.
2. Use your left hand on top of the foot for support.
3. Slowly rotate their foot out with your left hand while gliding (page 24) your right thumb toward the arch of their foot.
4. Repeat 3–5 times, and increase the pressure to their desire.

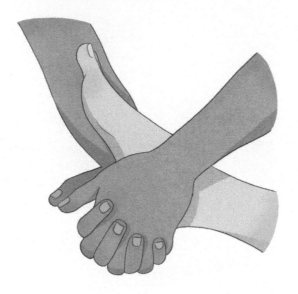

Heel Compression

The heels are one of the hardest places to add pressure. With this technique, you can successfully increase the pressure with little effort.

1. Add little to no oil or lotion to your hands.

2. Interlock your fingers, and place the heel of your palms on both sides of their ankle with your fingers facing down.

3. You can hold their ankle region for 20–30 seconds with moderate pressure, or slowly slide your palms down off their ankle and heel region 3–5 times, increasing the pressure to their desire.

Conclusion

Now you have the foundation to give incredible massages. You've learned about the many important systems of the body when it comes to massage and your important role as the giver as well as the receiver. Now that you know the basics of so many styles of massage, return to this book as often as you need. Prop it open and practice the styles that you love most on loved ones. Enjoy your continued journey into the wonderful, healing world of massage.

Resources

ASSOCIATIONS

Alliance for Massage Therapy Education (Massage Educators), AFMTE.org

American Massage Therapy Association (Insurance and Magazine), AMTAMassage.org

Associated Bodywork & Massage Professionals (Insurance and Magazine), ABMP.com

Massage Therapy Foundation (Research), MassageTherapyFoundation.org

BOOKS

Allen, Laura, LMBT. *Plain & Simple Guide to Therapeutic Massage & Bodywork Examinations.* LWW; 2nd edition, January 7, 2009.

Beck, Mark F. *Theory & Practice of Therapeutic Massage.* Milady; 5th edition, April 23, 2010.

Biel, Andrew. *Trail Guide to the Body: How to Locate Muscles, Bones and More.* Books of Discovery; 5th edition, November 6, 2014.

Fritz, Sandy, BS MS NCTMB. *Mosby's Fundamentals of Therapeutic Massage.* Mosby; 6th edition, April 4, 2016.

Fritz, Sandy. *Sports & Exercise Massage: Comprehensive Care for Athletics, Fitness, & Rehabilitation.* Mosby, 2013.

Lowe, Whitney W. LMT. *Orthopedic Massage: Theory and Technique.* Churchill Livingstone; 2nd edition, April 20, 2009.

Myers, Thomas W. *Anatomy Trains: Myofascial Meridians for Manual and Movement Therapists.* Churchill Livingstone; 3 edition, February 25, 2014.

Osborne, Carole, CMT NCBTMB. *Pre- and Perinatal Massage Therapy: A Comprehensive Guide to Prenatal, Labor, and Postpartum Practice.* LWW; 2nd edition, March 4, 2011.

Sohnen-Moe, Cherie M. *Business Mastery: A Guide for Creating a Fulfilling, Thriving Business and Keeping it Successful.* Sohnen-Moe Associates, Inc; 4th edition, January 1, 2008.

Thompson, Diana L. LMP. *Hands Heal: Communication, Documentation, and Insurance Billing for Manual Therapists.* LWW; 4th edition, July 5, 2011.

Upledger, John E. *Craniosacral Therapy.* Eastland Pr; 1st edition, February 1, 1983.

Werner, Ruth, LMP NCTMB. *A Massage Therapist's Guide to Pathology: Critical Thinking and Practical Application.* LWW; 6th edition, July 30, 2015.

WEBSITES

MassageToday.com
MassageMag.com

MASSAGE SUPPLIES

EarthLite.com
MassageWarehouse.com
CustomCraftworks.com
Bodyworkmall.com

ESSENTIAL OILS

WyndmereNaturals.com
NowFoods.com/essential-oils

References

Crane, Justin D., Daniel I. Ogborn, Colleen Cupido, Simon Melov, Alan Hubbard, Jacqueline M. Bourgeois, and Mark A. Tarnopolsky. "Massage Therapy Attenuates Inflammatory Signaling After Exercise-Induced Muscle Damage." *Science Translational Medicine.* 4, no. 119 (February 1, 2012): 119. DOI: 10.1126/scitranslmed.3002882.

Elliott, R. and B. Burkett, et al. "Massage Therapy as an Effective Treatment for Carpal Tunnel Syndrome." *Journal of Bodywork and Movement Therapy,* 17, no. 3 (July 2013): 332–8. DOI: 10.1016/j.jbmt.2012.12.003.

Field, Tiffany, Miguel Diego, and Maria Hernandez-Reif. "Potential Underlying Mechanisms for Greater Weight Gain in Massaged Preterm Infants." *Infant Behavior and Development,* 34, no. 3 (June, 2011): 383–389. DOI: 10.1016/j.infbeh.2010.12.001.

Jarmey, Chris and Gabiel Mojay. *Shiatsu: The Complete Guide.* London, UK: Thorsons, 1991.

Jensen M., M.N. Brant-Zawadzki, N. Obuchowski, M.T. Modic, D. Malkasian, and J.S. Ross. "Magnetic Resonance Imaging of the Lumbar Spine in People Without Back Pain." 2, no. 331 (July 14, 1994): 69–116. doi: 10.1056/NEJM199407143310201.

Lochtefeld, James G. *The Illustrated Encyclopedia of Hinduism: A-M.* New York, NY: The Rosen Publishing Group, 2001.

Morhenn, V., L.E. Beavin, and P.J Zak. "Massage Increases Oxytocin and Reduces Adrenocorticotropin Hormone in Humans." *Alternative Therapies in Health and Medicine,* 18, no. 6 (November-December 2012). ncbi.nlm.nih.gov/pubmed/23251939.

Novella, Steven. "What Is Traditional Chinese Medicine?" Accessed August 20, 2018. science-basedmedicine.org/what-is-traditional-chinese-medicine.

Perlman, A.I., A. Sabina, A.L. Williams, V.Y. Njike, and D.L. Katz. "Massage Therapy for Osteoarthritis of the Knee: A Randomized Controlled Trial." *Archives of Internal Medicine,* 166, no. 22 (December, 2006): 2533–8. DOI: 10.1001 /archinte.166.22.2533.

"Review Examines Clinical Trial Evidence on Complementary Approaches for Five Painful Conditions." National Center for Complementary and Integrative Medicine. Last modified: September 2, 2016. nccih.nih.gov/research /results/spotlight/five-painful-conditions.

Semple, David and Roger Smyth. *Oxford Handbook of Psychiatry.* 3rd ed. Oxford, UK: Oxford University Press, 2013.

Stergiou, Jemma. "Differences Between Eastern and Western Massage?" Accessed Aug. 20, 2018. www.keturah.com.au/blog /what-are-differences-between-eastern -and-western-massage.

Turan, N., and T.A. Aşt. "The Effect of Abdominal Massage on Constipation and Quality of Life." *Gastroenterology Nursing,* 39, no. 1 (January-February 2016): 48–59. DOI: 10.1097 /SGA.0000000000000202.

Index

Acknowledgements

First, I would like to thank my mom, Shirley Hoyme, for pushing me to go to massage school and my dad, Gary Hoyme, for believing in me. Thank you to my past students for inspiring me to always push myself to learn more. To my family—Yvette, Alexa, and Béa—thank you for putting up with my countless hours every week absorbed in learning more about massage. Thanks to Mary Jo Battey Otis for believing in me, being a great mentor, and pushing me harder to be a better massage therapist. A special thank you to my other mentors: Sharon Puszko, Lynda Solien-Wolfe, Laura Allen, Ruth Werner, Karen Kowal, Cherie Sohnen-Moe, Pete Whitridge, Ralph Stephens, Vivian Madison Mahoney, Michael McGillicuddy, Tracy Walton, and Sandy Fritz. Callisto Media, thank you for giving me this great opportunity to write this book. And finally, a big thank you to one of my past students (I still don't remember who it was!) for calling me a "massage nerd" in 2006. Your nickname caused me to buy the website domain the next day, and that started me on my incredible journey of www.MassageNerd.com.

About the Author

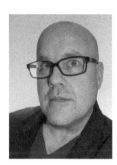

Ryan Jay Hoyme, LMT, BCTMB, is a board-certified massage therapist. He's worked in the health field for more than three decades and has practiced massage therapy for over two decades. He spent 14 years teaching massage to future practitioners, and continues to educate the community through his website and online videos. He is internationally known as the Massage Nerd and has won many awards in the massage industry. He's been inducted into the American and the International Massage Therapy Hall of Fame. Ryan has a large social media following and continues to be a role model and influencer.

MassageNerd.com

CPSIA information can be obtained
at www.ICGtesting.com
Printed in the USA
LVHW052142071118
596125LV00001B/1